THE INNATE DESIGN

IMPLEMENTING SELF-HEALING
TECHNIQUES FOR THE MODERN PATIENT

MELISSA AGUIRRE
AND
KYLE HOEDEBECKE, M.D.

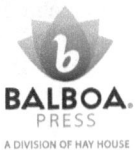

BALBOA.
PRESS

A DIVISION OF HAY HOUSE

Balboa Press books may be ordered through booksellers or by contacting:

Balboa Press
A Division of Hay House
1663 Liberty Drive
Bloomington, IN 47403
www.balboapress.com
1 (877) 407-4847

Because of the dynamic nature of the Internet, any web addresses or links contained in this book may have changed since publication and may no longer be valid. The views expressed in this work are solely those of the author and do not necessarily reflect the views of the publisher, and the publisher hereby disclaims any responsibility for them.

The author of this book does not dispense medical advice or prescribe the use of any technique as a form of treatment for physical, emotional, or medical problems without the advice of a physician, either directly or indirectly. The intent of the author is only to offer information of a general nature to help you in your quest for emotional and spiritual well-being. In the event you use any of the information in this book for yourself, which is your constitutional right, the author and the publisher assume no responsibility for your actions.

This work is nonfiction. However, some of the names and characteristics of the persons involved in case study or client cases have been changed in order to disguise their identities. Any resemblance to persons living or dead is pure coincidence and unintentional.

Any people depicted in stock imagery provided by Thinkstock are models, and such images are being used for illustrative purposes only.
Certain stock imagery © Thinkstock.

Print information available on the last page.

ISBN: 978-1-5043-6002-9 (sc)
ISBN: 978-1-5043-6003-6 (hc)
ISBN: 978-1-5043-6023-4 (e)

Library of Congress Control Number: 2016909707

Balboa Press rev. date: 07/25/2016

To each. To all. Let your conduct be a conduit of your message, let the love you give be an expression of your prayer, and let each day serve as curriculum. Listen to the wisdom of the body, your innate design, this magnificent blueprint to wellness and abundance wrapped in skin. Follow the road signs, yield for care, and be unabridged in your being knowing health is bona fide independence.

TABLE OF CONTENTS

Author's Note/ Preface...ix
Introduction...xi
Addressing Chronic Illness.. xv

1. Holism... 1
   What Are the Chakras?...3
   Key Yogic Tools for Healing 9

2. Root Chakra: Rooting Down to Rise Up 15
   Anxiety & Fear 16
   Addiction 23
   Eating Disorders 32
   Self Healing Tools...33

3. Sacral Chakra: Wellness is Movement...............................39
   Yoga and Trauma Recovery 41
   Self Healing Tools..48

4. Solar Plexus Chakra: Sourcing Your Power......................55
   Gut Brain 56
   IBS and Stress 59

Depression 60
Self Healing Tools 62

5. Heart Chakra: Love Thyself..................................71
   Stress and the Heart 73
   Fatigue/Burn Out...76
   High Blood Pressure and Yoga 79
   Self Healing Tools 81

6. Throat Chakra: Bridging Mind and Body.........89
   Power of Voice 91
   Sleep Apnea 92
   Thyroid and Throat Chakra 94
   Self Healing Tools 96

7. Third Eye Chakra: The Gem of Mentality 101
   Meditation 102
   Mindfulness 106
   Insomnia...113
   Self Healing Tools 119

8. Crown Chakra: Awakening to Wellness 121
   Making Meaning 122
   Prayer.. 125
   Self Healing Tools 125

9. Conclusion: Welcome Yourself Home................ 135

Yoga Pose Glossary 139
Index 155

AUTHOR'S NOTE/ PREFACE

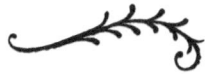

This book is an interdisciplinary collaboration between a yoga therapist and a physician who have witnessed the missing gap in allopathic medicine and are devoted to filling that gap with holistic, sustainable 'prescriptions' to patients. As they have both witnessed these modalities, practices, and lifestyle choices be more effective on the healing of their patients, Melissa and Kyle wanted to find a way to reach more individuals to inform, inspire, and influence people of our time to generate an effective way to prevent illness and care for patients of the future.

Many conclusions drawn from this book are derived from experience and personal understanding based off of patient interaction, case study, and current research being done in alternative and holistic medicine. As we navigate through these holistic modalities, the hope is to suggest each practice as an adjunction to therapy and to be adopted into daily life style choices.

INTRODUCTION

Over the past decade, an abundance of alternative and complementary practices have become widely accessible to the public and are slowly becoming integrated into our current healthcare system. This book is a tool for healthcare professionals and patients to provide a holistic perspective when treating and working with patients in addition to those individuals who want to learn more about this aspect of healing.

Although "Do No Harm" is not specifically stated in the Hippocratic Oath, medical providers understand and yield to the ethical principles of first doing no harm. With an ever-increasing dependency of drug interventions and surgical procedures, doctors are straying further away from facilitating overall patients' health, wellness, and quality of life (QOL). Rather, patients are experiencing much less healing and more dependency and stagnation. The current procedures and regulations of healthcare are no longer keeping people accountable for their health, but addressing patients simply as chemical processes; therefore, treating patients with other chemical processes. This cycle has caused more illnesses, debt, and disease. When the definition of health is the absence of disease and/or injury, it compresses the value and experience of life into a limited continuum. This book will offer a larger scale of what health really is through individual flourishing not mechanically - but holistically. We will provide a new paradigm for healthcare professionals to use when consulting patients and assisting them through prevention and recovery. The objective is to move away from the sole utilization of the biomedical model and into addressing the whole person including lifestyle, environment, spirituality, and nutrition to instill a healthier, happier QOL. Understanding the Chakra system gives medical providers an effective model to counsel their patients on how to better internalize locus of control- making choices that are cost effective which will lead to healing and flourishing.

According the Centers of Disease Control (CDC) roughly 75% of healthcare spending goes to treating preventable diseases. Rather than operating healthcare as disease control, addressing patients as a whole to counsel them according to imbalances in their lifestyle and choices so that patients can empower themselves into sustainable healing and illness prevention. Educating oneself on mindfulness-based trainings and exploring the Chakra system provides a new pathway to healing and improved health.

We must take action and change our current system as, according to the Institute of Medicine, 30% of health care cost (roughly $750 billion annually) are wasted and do not improve health. Much of this waste comes from the focus on sub-specialization in medicine and skyrocketing healthcare costs not correlated to outcomes. An unproportionate, excessive amount of money is spent on the last months of life to increase quantity rather than QOL Furthermore, fears of lawsuits also drive medical providers to perform numerous unwarranted tests and additional spending.

The purpose of this book is to provide health care professionals and patients with a broader, intuitive lens in addressing a more participatory medical practice. Implementing new modalities that refine the patient/ doctor relationship so patients are seen, met, and understood by their medical team allowing for an improved clarity leading to sustainable healing.

Unfortunately, the medical culture is saturated with over-medicating patients. In addition to potential side effects and interactions between medications, many of these pills do not correct the problem itself. Furthermore, many pathologies can be attributed to imbalances in chakras. With a direct correlation between the 7 main chakras and the neuroendocrine system, this model boasts many cost effective, holistic ways of improving healing.

This book is a collaboration between Dr. Kyle Hoedebecke and Yoga Therapist Melissa Aguirre to merge westernized medicine with holistic, natural modalities based off of experience and observation in patient healing and wellness. Within these pages compose both evidence-based research and case studies that point to self-sustainability in hopes to raise awareness and show the importance of accountability in healing and health care. This book does not take the place of the care of primary care providers or specialists - rather is intended to allow the reader to evaluate health from a new perspective and integrate non pharmacological treatments as a source of health and healing.

ADDRESSING CHRONIC ILLNESS

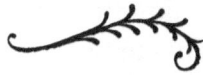

"The doctor of the future will give no medicine, but will instruct his patient in the care of the human frame, in diet, and in the cause and prevention of disease." —Thomas Edison (1902)

The problem of chronic illness drains the medical system, and the current models show minimal productivity in resolving this issue. As our nation continues to hemorrhage money for preventable medical expenses, providers and patients must look for an alternative approach to bridge the gap between conventional and integrative health for a direction in our healthcare system. Primary-care providers have become exhausted and overwhelmed, leading to burnout within our medical professional and caregiver communities. Integrative health proposes the potential of restoring the joy to medical practices while watching people heal as a solution to the epidemic of serving the chronically ill.

Many specific chronic conditions often correlate with lifestyle choices. Examples include diagnoses such as stroke, arthritis, heart disease, some cancers, diabetes, and obesity. Physicians recommend regular physical activity throughout the week to help prevent the above-mentioned pathologies. In addition to other exercises, regularly practicing yoga and being mindful of lifestyle choices offers a great way to help ward off these conditions and improve one's overall physical and mental health, thereby offering an augmented quality of life (QOL).

Lifestyle choice has a huge influence over one's potential of being diagnosed with a chronic illness. It also plays a vital role in the chakra modality. Although some chronic illnesses are a result of aging, economic resources, or genetics, one has a better chance of preventing a chronic illness by paying attention to healthy diet, avoidance of tobacco products, and regular exercise. This information is nothing new, so we must find ways to derail dysfunctional lifestyle choices and replace them with new positive choices. With knowledge comes responsibility, and your first step is to empower yourself to take control of your health. You need to also realize that it is possible to live a vibrant, peaceful life.

Mahatma Gandhi once said, "A man is but the product of his thoughts. What he thinks, he becomes." When we efficiently absorb the tools and wisdom into who we are, we can generate the person we want to be. Even if you are living with a chronic illness, the effect of that illness can be limited with lifestyle choices. Whether it be physically or by adopting a new attitude of peace by pursuing practices and eating habits that strive to nourish the whole body—just as you are, both can have an impact on your health. This is a solution-oriented book that will provide practical ways to implement exercises into your daily routine, help you cultivate a new craving of feeling well, and release old habits that serve no positive purposes.

Let's get started!

HOLISM

Health is a large word. It embraces not the body only, but the mind and spirit as well; and not today's pain or pleasure alone, but the whole being and outlook of man. —James H. West

The chakra system is rooted in holism, the concept that the entire person should be addressed to include psychological, spiritual, emotional, mental, and lifestyle factors. Applying holistic practices broadens both the provider's and patient's healing capacity in conventional, alternative, and complementary medicine, so as to enrich the scope of medical practices to optimize a patient's health potential. Holism encompasses occupational environment, lifestyle habits, mental processes, psychological factors, and other experiences that influence one's state of being.

Specifically, the chakra system serves as a holistic model that expounds and directs the influence of all quadrants within the patient's life. For example, an individual may suffer from chronic back pain, even though all medical exams and imaging modalities have shown no evidence of pathology. Holism allows the health practitioner to apply a wider lens of evaluation and treatment for this complaint. Whether due to stress or dysfunctional postural habits, one can better advise the patient in cost-effective, holistic practices rather than immediately turning to surgical interventions or oral painkillers.

Holism also addresses how each part of the body influences one's entire being. In Jon Kabat-Zinn's *Full Catastrophe Living*, he talks about interconnectedness and wholeness throughout the body:

> It is a universe in itself [our body], consisting of more than 10 trillion cells that all ultimately derive from one single cell, organized into tissues and organs and systems and structures, with a built-in ability to regulate itself as a whole to maintain internal balance and order down to the nano level of interacting molecular structures. In a word, our bodies are undeniably self-organizing and self-healing at every level you care to look at ... All these are highly integrated, interconnected regulatory processes operating through elaborate feedback loops.

Our biology is interconnected and self-regulated, meaning that any single piece can positively or negatively affect the entire body. Numerous experiences in our day-to-day living exemplify this theory, such as when we feel sad, we may not have an appetite, or when we are under chronic stress, our bodies may break out in a rash. Our minds and bodies share a sphere of experience, each mirroring the other. Science has validated much of what the ancient yogis have taught in reference to the mind-body connection.

What Are the Chakras?

We are no animals. We are galaxies with skin. —Tara Sophia Mohr

Dating back to 1750–500 BCE, chakras derived from the Vedic culture known for the Vedas, the oldest scriptures of Hinduism. Many holistic practices are products of this culture, which includes theories of awakening, intuitional practice, as well as the belief that the individual is a realization of the self. The chakras are simply an organic formula for the individual to use to become pure or to rebalance in the body.

Chakras—meaning *wheel* or *circle* in Sanskrit—are psychospiritual vortices of energy within and surrounding the body. Though many exist, we will focus on the seven main chakras within the body. With that in mind, the idea is that humans manifest from an interplanetary system. For example, the saying "as within, so without" means that the elements of the planet are the same as those within the body itself. The element *water* is illustrated in the body as fluid, urine, and other unsolidified components: the element *earth* is illustrated in the body as bone structure, skin, and other physical configurations; *fire* is demonstrated through body temperature, digestion, and other metabolizing apparatuses; and *air* is exhibited through respiration, gas, and participates in digestion. Therefore, the Vedic culture believed the human being exists as a fractal of the universe. They used yoga practice and holistic interventions to clean and balance the elements, which would, therefore, clean and balance the system.

The chakras utilize movement, touch, voice, mind, and lifestyle choice to influence anatomical, physiological, and psychological development. They delineate how depending on external influences and choice will yield catalysts to psychophysical expansion or malady in the body. Each chakra expounds glandular reactions with the brain producing *tendencies* in the human. The yogis identified fifty tendencies associated with different glands throughout the body.

The processes needed to balance the chakras are associated with practices such as meditation, chanting/singing, diet, lifestyle choice, ethics, yoga, and service. Each chakra has specific practices relating to both the neuroendocrine system and psychophysical relationship with the body to influence the specific region it correlates with. As there have been many evidence-based yoga practices that support, prevent, and rehabilitate ailments or injuries, the science behind yoga poses and their effects on the body is ample. Repeating yoga poses or movement patterns puts sustained pressure on key areas throughout the body. These positions also affect the flow of blood and lymphatic fluid throughout the circulatory system. As the body moves through functional patterns, this process helps optimize neuromuscular pathways that decrease discomfort in the body, making it easier for the person to function and live a flourishing life.

Overall, the chakras acknowledge that different people are at different places in their development. This knowledge allows the physician to identify what the patient is facing, thereby offering a better way to meet the patient where he or she is. For the individual, the chakras show up to delineate where the person should work on to enhance his or her own evolution and wellness.

The Chakra Story

When you touch the celestial in your heart, you will realize that the beauty of your soul is so pure, so vast and so devastating that you have no option but to merge with it. You have no option but to feel the rhythm of the universe in the rhythm of your heart. —Amit Ray

The chakras were utilized as a method of returning to a balanced state, or as the Vedic tradition says, "returning to the beloved." They applied the chakras as a lens to discover aspects that were unbalanced within the body. They accessed the chakras through yoga, meditation, breath work, and lifestyle choices to self-correct and heal the imbalances.

The structure of the chakras is demonstrated through realization with this tradition exemplifying how an imbalance secondary to trauma, suffering, grief, and stress may allow one to realize him- or herself. This happens through the Vedic's desire to merge with God or self-purification; thus, removing impurities from the body on psychological, spiritual, physical, emotional, and mental levels is required for balance and health.

The first chakra, known as the *root chakra*, begins as a delineation of the average, mundane life. This is where one simply *exists* in a monotonous manner characterized by survival, autopilot, and stability. This space represents one's potential and acknowledges that people vary in their development. This reveals what people can improve upon within themselves to become better and create more purpose.

From this space, one experiences *transformation* and moves upward to the second or *sacral chakra,* which is affected by a trauma or any experience that interrupts the average, mundane life. Change, loss, suffering, or trauma may force the individual to move outside his or her comfort zone and experience unfamiliar emotions or contemplations in relationship with life.

The third chakra, the solar plexus chakra, alchemizes the experience of trauma or change - either causing the person to become defeated from the experience or increasingly more motivated and inspired by such experience. Personal transformation occurs from the developed inspiration. Once the discomfort is functionally alchemized it moves upwards.

The fourth chakra, known as the the *heart chakra*, serves as a location of self-understanding where one decides "what is and isn't me" so as to set healthy boundaries based on previous experiences of discomfort. From here, one begins to practice service to others and healthy boundaries instilling clarity and balance in emotions and contemplations. This state - elicited from one's experiences - moves through the chest up into the fifth chakra, the throat chakra.

The throat chakra encompasses one's ability to express themselves and that which they stand. Creativity and connection manifests here as one becomes more in tune with his or her surroundings. The throat chakra is a place of self-actualization acting as a bridge between the emotional mind and spirit manifesting up into the sixth chakra, the third eye center.

The third eye maintains a relationship with the body's command center in the form of the hypothalamus and pituitary gland which instills an inner knowledge to have the ability to experience intuitive relationships with life and a cultivation of wisdom. Wisdom is the manifestation of healed pain that finally flourishes here in the sixth chakra allowing one to extend compassion and counsel to others, along with developing psycho-spiritual awareness.

With this newly found spiritual cognizance one moves upward to the seventh chakra, known as the crown chakra where the individual experiences a spiritual connection. This is what the Vedic's truly desired. The physiognomies that he or she experiences are surrender, trusting in divine providence, and separation being dissipated. The Vedic culture viewed this as the space of oneness and philosophical concepts.

This elusive description of the chakra story is simply an expression of how the Vedic culture applied the experience of returning to balance in the body and how external influences correlate with internal factors. Applying this model assists the health practitioner in identifying an initial focal point of self-treatment with the patient based on where the patient is in his or her life. The chakra model is a great way to identify where patients are located on the continuum so they may develop within their own personal story leading to self-sustainable wellness.

A Medical and Developmental Lens

Although the chakras come from a philosophical-religious tradition, there appears to be a potential role in the medical realm due to the interdependence of the neuroendocrine system and cognition. These connections represent a relatively new idea in neuroscience research. The major chakras discussed in the story above are directly associated with the neuroendocrine system in addition to serving as mental/emotional centers. The chakras themselves are not physical entities and cannot be held or examined like an object, but exist solely as energy and hold a strong relationship with the physical functioning of our body. Influencing hormones and the body's organization of health, they communicate through fascia tissue. The seven major Chakras are comprised of centers of hormone production or high concentrations of gap junction cells - serving as intercellular networks that allow for rapid signal transfer throughout various parts of the body.

Gap junctions are responsible for many of the transmission of signals required for medications to take effect. [62] Unfortunately some have also shown to block gap junction channels, which can lead to unwanted or secondary effects.[63] One known negative effect that can occur naturally or artificially is called the "bystander effect." When an injured cell receives a signal to die gap junctions may send the same messages to adjacent cells. This can cause the otherwise unaffected healthy bystander cells to also die.[64] Gap junctions do not only provide negative signals as they may also serve a role in wound healing.[79][80] Specifically, gap junctions may serve to electrically and chemically link cells throughout the body of almost all animals including humans. They are extremely important in the function of cardiac muscle where gap junctions serve to allow the heart to beat by creating a contraction and causing subsequent forward blood flow. Our entire nervous system relies on gap junctions often referred to as an electrical synapse. These connections connect our brain to the rest of our body and allow for nearly instantaneous signal transfer. In the eye, nerve cells within the retina demonstrate large numbers of gap junctions - playing a part in light and color perceptions.

The human body and its systematic interconnections are all joined by the theory of holism as well as through the gap junction interface. As the chakras are not a physical entity, we observe them through cell-to-cell communication and the interactions with the nervous and endocrine systems. When we observe the embryological process in the womb, we see how the chakras influence our beings starting in the developmental stages. They manifest and help coordinate activity as the embryological process begins with multiplication of cells and separation into different cell types or layers. This rapid division and differentiation occurs through chemical signals transferred by gap junctions. As this process continues, the primitive spinal cord also forms - thereby supporting even more rapid electronic and chemical movement and messaging. These transmissions are needed for proper growth and development from undifferentiated cells into the specialized organs of the body. As we see the chakras, though not an organ system, physically exist within areas of high gap junction cell concentration, it is no surprise how much we are impacted by this system.

It is fascinating to observe the role of the chakras in development physically, spiritually, and psychologically. The first chakra relates to the formation of the physical development; hence why it is so rooted in survival and physical comfort. It is here that we begin to discover our right to exist and our right to survive. The second chakra is attributed to more movement and sensation which correlates to the first three years of our life when we are still dependent upon our mother but explore the distinctions between good and bad or pleasure and pain. Psychologically we develop our emotional experience and relationship with the world generating our right to feel. The following years age four to ten are developed in relationship to the third chakra developing ego and connecting with our power. This stage may hold the desire to 'please' others while also developing independence to self create and self define where the shadow of the third also begins to surface which is to feel shame or inadequacy. The child is beginning to process experiences to create will and purpose rooting into the right to act and choose.

By ages ten through fourteen, psychological development exists more in social context and is based upon the right to be loved and love or the right to feel accepted and accept which is sourced by the fourth chakra. These concepts have always been underlain but now are being actualized and the individual is much more aware of these experiences. At this point we have picked up on social cues that influence our relationship with others and how we hold relationship with ourselves in the social scheme where we begin to move into initiative and alchemize the power from the third chakra. The fifth chakra is the manifestation of voice and creative expression. Ages fourteen through eighteen hold the key for this development as one begins to express who they are and explore the meaning of the human experience. This influences the craving to do something that contributes to the world and others along with affirming the right to be heard and speaking in truth.

The sixth and seventh chakra coexist in adulthood. This is the knowledge of recognizing patterns and creating deeper meaning moving into the pursuit of knowing and awakening. Although our entire life we bounce up and down the chakra continuum, this developmental process is where we create and experience the discovery and actualization of the chakra components in relationship with our being. The one thing that must be comprehended about the chakras is that they are not physical vortices spinning in our bodies, they are simply an energetic force influencing over our experience, viewpoints, and relationship with living. These spaces give us an understanding of our psychology and how external elements and thought platforms influence our ability to live in suffering or, alternatively, in health.

Key Yogic Tools for Healing

"I have been a seeker and I still am, but I stopped asking the books and the stars. I started listening to the teaching of my Soul." ~ by Rumi

An explanation to understanding imbalances is exemplified by a state of having too much or too little. Balance is a condition in which elements are equal or in optimal proportion. The same principle applies to the chakras and is theoretically simple. A chakra may hold too much energy and be excessive. For example, the third chakra relates to our power center so an excess would look like tyranny. In order to balance, one must discharge that energy or implement attitudes of compassion and humility. Just like when something is too hot, then we cool it down. A chakra may hold too little energy and be weak. For example, a deficient third chakra may present as depression. In order to rebalance, one must create meaning and action to stimulate the flow of energy. Just like when someone is sick he or she must receive care and nourishment. Each imbalance can be addressed with validation by acknowledgement, clarity by direction, physically by bodywork and movement, spiritually through faith, prayer, and meditation, emotionally by processing experiences and feelings, music, creativity, and application of lifestyle choice.

Balancing chakras means addressing the imbalances in one's existence that present in the mental, spiritual, emotional, psychological, environmental, or physical realms. By learning the chakra modality it creates an understanding of both the nature and function of that particular chakra. One can digest it through reflecting on his or her own personal experiences related to the chakras and the imbalances that are exposed, thus, implementing practices that create new neural pathways on a cellular level influencing habits and our relationships to ourselves and the world to maintain balance and optimal health.

Balancing the chakras are associated with practices such as meditation, chanting/singing, diet, lifestyle choice, ethics, yoga, and service. Each chakra has specific practices relating to the neuroendocrine system and psychophysical relationship with the body to influence the specific region it correlates with.

Integrating these different practices derives from the yogic tradition that instills balancing and healing in the body, mind, and spirit. Because the yogic philosophy sees the body as three separate entities existing as a whole. The human experience is a collaborative effort generated by mind, body, and spirit, therefore, yoga was created as an effective way to preserve unity knowing that the part affects the whole. The first yogic tool in healing the body through the chakra modality begins with asana or poses consisting of stretching, strengthening and movement. Because the body and mind interact as two interwoven domains, the poses connect different areas of the body and, therefore, often influencing more than one chakra. This is similar to how gap junctions link cells throughout the body.

As many yoga poses move through the body's synergistic functioning, a pose may positively influence more than just the targeted imbalance. The organized movement has a holistic impact within the body compatible with the body's strive for homeostasis. This is why yoga is a timeless healing technology.

Asana (Yoga Posture)

As there have been many evidence-based yoga practices that support, prevent and rehabilitate ailments or injuries, the science behind yoga poses and their effects the body is ample. Repeating yoga poses or movement patterns put sustained pressure on key areas throughout the body. These positions also affect the flow of blood and lymphatic fluid throughout the circulatory system. As the body moves through functional patterns, this process helps optimize neuromuscular pathways that decrease discomfort in the body making it easier for the person to function and live a flourishing life.

Mindfulness and Meditation

Mindfulness is the innate ability of tuning into the details of your experience with each present moment and may show up through the way you nourish your body, participate in relationships, and celebrate each moment of your life - all in the simplicity of being present. Mindfulness is a basic human capacity of paying attention to the present moment with intention in a non-judging way. Meditation is an opportunity to tune into yourself and experience it in stillness, provoking one to touch base with what lies beneath the story, beneath the circumstances, beneath or tribulations. The practice of simply being, rather than doing.

Pranayama (Breathing Exercises)

Our breath is central to life - without it we do not exist. Pranayama exercises are practices that change the breath pace or techniques of organized inhaling and exhaling. Each type is used for a different purpose from slowing the mind, generating clarity, or stimulating energy.

Personal development

Personal development manifests through the process of self-exploration. Each chakra proposes specific keys to focus on moving through in order to attain balance. For example, the influence of the yoga practice may inspire one to eat mindfully and in moderation such as choosing foods that are more nourishing rather than a standard meals provided at fast food restaurants. The physical movements and goal towards wellness can open one into a new habit of thinking positively and instilling patience; thus, improving many areas of that individual's life by feeling an overall sense of peace and happiness.

Ethics

Ethics are built upon boundaries and what becomes important to the individual. Ethics establish a framework for the individual to feel a greater sense of purpose by the limits set and the ability to uphold integrity aligned with what is valued for that individual.

Service to Others

Often times, I consult with clients who feel unfulfilled in their work routines and daily lives because of the belief that they are not contributing to the world or helping others. Service is therapeutic to our existence because we are a collective of beings who share this Earth and when we do good for one another we reap psychological and emotional benefits. You can read more on this in the fourth chakra chapter.

Intention and Affirmation

Intention spawns in the mind and sets the tone of how we live. It is a form of asking, a form of choosing, and a form of living. Intention setting is the first step in creating the exemplary life one would want. Affirmation - or mantra - is the process of reminding what we already know. "I will be calm" is an example of how one can remind the body of its own capacity to calm and the ability to purposefully choose to remain so. Beginning the day to set an intention and affirming that notion will construct the day upon that experience. Intention and affirmation have the power to structure our perception in a way where peace or wellness is our natural state. Through practice and the maintenance of intention, we can find resilience and insight each day. This serves well for those who suffer from stress, anxiety, or other ailments. There is a reason the saying 'attitude is everything' exists. As clique as it is, it is genuine. This practice helps set a habit to release dysfunctional attitudes and perspectives in order to generate a healthy outlook and temperament.

All of these practices have been selectively 'prescribed' for balancing each chakra for different physical ailments and psycho-spiritual imbalances.

ROOT CHAKRA

Rooting Down to Rise Up

~~~~~~

"We root down to rise up."

The root chakra is the first of the chakras located in the coccygeal plexus found in the pelvic floor region. A function for the root chakra correlates with urophysis, a discrete structure, found at the base of the spinal cord that produces neuropeptides that help control water and electrolyte balances, blood pressure, and smooth muscle contractions. Muladhara is the Sanskrit word for this chakra meaning "root support." With so many nerves located here, much of our natural instincts emulate from this place. This is also the location from which our rudimentary desires derive - survival, physical desires, mental wishes, psycho-spiritual yearnings (i.e. moral and righteous), and liberation. This chakra can see where we can grow and acknowledge where we stand on the path of own personal development. A visual metaphor comes from the idea of the nervous system as the plant and the brain as the flower - making the first chakra imperative because nothing can flourish without its roots. Here lies the fertile ground for consciousness to grow.

Additionally, the first chakra has other characteristics traditionally associated with this location such as solid, firm, clear, autopilot, color of a golden sun, "I am," and one's overall potential. The idea that we come from bliss-making emotional balances the ways to achieve bliss - from where the imbalances such as selfishness, resistance to change, and addiction come. On a psychophysical level, a balanced root chakra expounds discipline, self control, physical strength, and patience.

A good analogy of the first chakra is that of a seed. Each one of us contains an intelligent blueprint for entelechy or a realization of potential within each of us. Our life journey is the process of actualizing our entelechy, but when we do not progress or make choices to nourish ourselves our entelechy becomes blocked. A seed that lands on a desolate surface in an environment unsuitable for taking root and providing sustenance doesn't grow. However, when the seed grounds on a foundation bearing the requisites to flourish, it may easily take root and be nourished. Likewise, our potential can only be attained if we are supporting ourselves in ways to prosper mentally, physically, emotionally, and spiritually. To continue with this analogy, a seed must be buried beneath the dirt to thrive. Therefore, each experience - both negative and positive - that may bury us, even in the darkness, still creates the potential for us to unlock our own entelechy to yield an profound, abundant life.

Anxiety & Fear

Personal experience has shown that about 85% of clients experience anxiety, stress, or hold large amounts of fear in relation to the future and their lives. It is no surprise that anxiety plagues this world because most people do not take time to ground and care for themselves. Many feel there is never enough time or experience and inadvertent underlying form of self-sabotage is running rampant through their lives. We live in a scarcity-based society that bombard us with messages of 'not enough money', 'not enough time', 'not enough', and 'never enough'. This conditions our thinking to consistently feeling lack and can develop into a chronic experience of not being supported or provided for, thus, giving birth to fear and anxiety disorders.

The antidotes to anxiety and fear are abundance, courage, clarity, and confidence. Because life happens through us, not to us; we can begin to realize our ability to be in control of our relationship to the circumstance. You may read this again through the book as this principle is concrete to alleviating suffering; you yourself are not your circumstances, challenges, or problems. Your identity is not defined by those things, nor the depiction others may create. The moment you begin to define yourself as such, you become a victim of your experiences and you give your power away. Stop doing that! We get so lost in giving away our power to fear and anxiety or situations we have no control over that we lose sight of our ability to feel at peace and trust in the curriculum of our lives.

Abundance
"I am enough."

The formula of abundance comes from asking and trusting. Affirmation as well as mantras consist of how we can ask for things in our lives. Through prayer or affirmation - 'I am intelligent', 'I am unique' - we begin to manifest our reality. When we think in lack, we receive in lack. Everything begins with our viewpoint of the world. Many do not realize that a negative point of view can block life's blessings. We must slow down in order to receive our blessings. These thought platforms are cultivated through redundant belief in illusion or fear or the story we created. If we say we are not good enough, we affirm a reality where we are not good enough. Our thoughts alone can keep us stuck and are the catalyst to self sabotage. By practicing self care and creating space between our thoughts and our reactions, we begin to inquire about what is real and what isn't.

Slowing down is essential to awakening to the truth. You are supported and held if you believe it. Action is the only witness to belief. We must live in obedience to the truth and use our actions to depict that trust. If we are behaving as though we live in lack or the latter of contributing nothing to the visions we may have or the hopes we create- then all that is left is lack and nothing. We must act in accordance. We must be convicted by the word and step into abundance. It is so easy to get caught up in the longing that we miss out on the opportunities to be blessed and be present. The quality of each moment is measured by the volume of our presence. We must show up in order for abundance to be met.

Another concept we must understand about abundance is that when abundance is present, resistance will always show up. Similar to when there is light, there is darkness. When this discomfort arises, it is easy to stop and hide. Resistance is affirmation shouting you are exactly where you need to be. The feeling of discomfort is natural. Be mindful of survival mode kicking in and invite a pause. When we pause to observe the discomfort and move into it, abundance will flow. It is through these dualities that enhance the potential of the other. Let the resistance be stair steps to abundance. Each moment presents a choice- for us to live abundantly in each present moment. Or to fret anytime resistance surfaces, buy into the illusion, and live frustrated, longing for something more. Choose abundance.

Courage
"I am strong and resilient."

Fear is a survival mechanism embedded into our being that is designed to protect us from environmental threats. Many individuals share their fears and conclude the experience with statements such as, "Once I overcome the fear, then I will." or "Once I get over my fear, then I can change." The truth about fear is nobody ever 'overcomes' it. We must accept this and the reason behind that comes from the fact that fear is so fine tuned into our existence as a survival instinct that it proves nearly impossible to completely flush from our lives. It serves to protect us and we can hold gratitude towards this sensation rather than frustration or shame. This is how we begin to move through fear.

Naturally, when we experience discomfort, avoidance begins to surface and can lead to paralysis from moving through the obstacle. Courage, however, is the antidote to fear and manifests through showing up and meeting your fear. Simply showing up to observe and witness begins the process of redirecting your experience and reactions. Wellness can be described by the word movement. Movement is the catalyst to change, to energy, and to action. So many people allow their fears to hold them hostage, but when one simply generates the courage to reflect upon it, one will then discover that the dramatic emotions created by fear are really propelled by illusion and self sabotage that inhibits wellness. We procrastinate or invent excuses to justify the lack of movement in our lives feeding into the illusion that we are content when really one is afraid of change or taking accountability for life. This also plays into the fear of letting go. Sometimes the pain of holding on and being dragged constantly by the imbalance, the toxic individual, the bad environment - or whatever it is - can be more painful than the initial sting of finally letting go and taking power back.

The act of courage through acknowledging fear begins an entire journey of moving towards a more resilient and refined existence. When fear arises, our first instinct is to run - and that is natural - but this reaction is responsible for so many shattered dreams, relationships, and health imbalances. Anxiety, discouragement, and overly thinking plagues our minds when we move into avoidance from the discomfort that stagnates. If we take action to step into it wholeheartedly, knowing we will either fall (which never feels good, but is so temporary) and learn a lesson or we will fly and yield abundance.

Clarity
"I hold vision and direction for myself."

As people, we are filled by a collection of desires, experiences, likes, and dislikes that manifest into our sense of that which we want and that which we don't. However, this collection may feel like a maze of constant unknowing at times. When we are lost in this labyrinth, our thinking becomes discombobulated to the point where we cannot even articulate that which we want or need in the moment. A lack of clarity leads to sensations of being overwhelmed and anxiety that create this underlying feeling of inadequacy so we do not impact or change ourselves. Clarity is a form of insight that the mind and body needs in order to flourish in the present.

In our culture, entertainment and media constantly invade us with messages of what we should want, do, or who we should be. In reality, we are all individually unique expressions of ourselves and we distort who we are and what we want when we buy into these expectations. This is where grounding and creating space come into play. It is okay not to know all the answers and to not know entirely who you are because our entire life is an evolution of self actualization. We are expected at such a young age to decide what we want to do with our lives and so many people give themselves away to things that take their power, identity, and joy due to societal or familial pressures.

The first step to clarity is grounding, or the rooting into the present moment. Direct your attention to your vitality - your breath, warmth, and the physical sensations you feel. Journaling or creating lists are excellent ways to see how you feel and what you want. Dissect this list and then take action to move into those things you desire or need in your life. It is not always easy to remain accountable to the things we love and the things that serve us. However, if we neglect our self care, the repercussions could wreck our health and our peace. We cannot serve from an empty vessel. Routine and structure generate the conduit to show up for ourselves and others. Consistency in our wellness is imperative. Without the maintenance, imbalance will surface once again. A plant cannot flourish unless it is rooted. What makes us any different?

Overwhelm and lack clarity are also a repercussion of not creating space. Space is clarity. I always recommend meditation, but if not a mindful practice is it your environment? Take time to go places that ground and relax you so you can generate clarity. Is it someone in your life? It may not be that you have to completely release the relationship but you can create space. In our culture, we suffocate under schedules, expectations, and tasks. We create so much pressure on ourselves where we can't even breathe so we just avoid. In coming, we will discuss more on mindfulness and meditation. These practices shift the brain at a cellular level making it more natural to create space- if not physically, then mentally.

A Medical Lens

There are many medical pathologies attributed to the root chakra due to the presence of the coccygeal plexus, urophysis correlation, and surrounding structures. Medical providers familiar with the pelvis can attest to the multiple potential pathologies that may occur within this area of the body. This is one of the reasons why the exact diagnosis for pelvic pain may prove challenging for providers and patients alike. We will delve into a few of the specific pathologies attributes to the root chakra imbalances and evaluate the medical reasoning behind these connections.

The coccygeal plexus consists of components of the S4, S5, and coccygeal nerves. These nerves play an important role in pelvic floor function. One aspect is through the bladder and control of urination. Weakness in the urethral sphincters, from childbirth or other causes, will lead to unintended or uncontrolled urine leakages. One can compensate for these weaknesses through pelvic floor strengthening as seen with Kegel exercises or other pelvic floor training.

There are many other diagnoses involving pelvic pain or dysfunction attributed to the Root chakra due to their co-location. Pathology in the hips and lower spinal cord may create stenosis of the nerve canals or even cause inappropriate spinal curvatures. Compression of the lumbar/sacral nerves can cause localized lower back or hip pain. Under certain conditions, this can cause lower extremity weakness or radiating pain can be felt in the buttocks or lower extremities as seen with nerve compression.

Sexual and urinary dysfunction as well are affected. Kidney stones can cause intense pelvic pain and lead to more significant medical issues like infection and urinary retention. Interstitial cystitis is also a common cause of chronic pelvic pain associated with urination. Poor circulation or nerve signaling can lead to impotence and sexual dysfunction.

The gastrointestinal tract is also attributed to this chakra. One of the most common causes of pelvic pain caused many GI concerns are constipation and diverticulitis. Improved water and fiber intake as well as increased physical activity can help improve symptoms and regularity. These can also help more severe GI pathologies such as, ulcerative colitis or Crohn's disease, to augment treatment from specialists.

Lastly, problems with root chakra relate to poor coping mechanisms utilized in an attempt to heal this location via poor coping mechanisms. Poor diet, sex, alcohol, and drugs - among other behaviors - can be used in excess in a failed attempt to heal. By searching out and engaging positive healing techniques, the individual may truly find a healthy method in which to initiate a return to health.

There are many other pathologies traditionally attributed to this chakra: Addiction (alcohol, sex, cocaine), anxiety disorders, mental health, anorexia, depression, learning disorders, hemorrhoids, hypertension (chemicals from urophysis), weight gain/loss, skin disorders (rashes), migraines, psoas/internal muscle problems, and resistance to change. By understanding our developmental status, sourcing what the underlying imbalance is- a simple shift in thinking or postural correction can make all the difference. Practicing preventive medicine begins at the root chakra, otherwise, when derailed the risk for above pathologies is increased.

Addiction

**"Please keep in mind the distinction
between treatment and healing: treatment
originates from outside where healing
comes from within." Dr. Andrew Weil**

Addiction is an epidemic that reaches beyond substance abuse and can even be reflected through caffeine, sugar, behavioral, and many other habits. Most people exhibit some degree of addiction to something. Though some have far more severe repercussions than others, addiction is the product of a society or culture that embodies scarcity and extreme expectations. They may manifest from a sensation of survival mode or security, but constructing the focus to rebuilding neurological deficits in healing the dysfunction begins by addressing the pain for why people experience addiction. Our behavior is never really about the substance, rather about the underlying imbalance that is stimulated by the addiction in the first place - such as adverse childhood events, trauma, self sabotage, and others.

Currently, a huge treatment gap exists between addiction and recovery. A 2009 study showed that twenty-three million Americans age twelve and older suffer from alcohol and drug addictions while less than ten percent actually receive treatment. Furthermore, forty to sixty percent of drug addicts will relapse at least once from their treatment plan. This gap exists because either treatment is too expensive, the addict is not ready to receive recovery, there are access barriers, or even the stigma around recovery may sway addicts away from seeking help.

There is a need to integrate cost effective and sustainable treatment modalities into modern health care that address the underlying cause of addiction and suitable treatments tailored to the individual. As allopathic medicine has limitations in who and where it can reach, holistic modalities may exist deeply in addiction prevention and rehabilitation as it is oriented around addressing all components to one's life.

Going on her 30th year of sobriety at age 70, Sue could not have more vitality. Turning to God and asking for guidance directs her closer to her commitment to sobriety and sharing her experiences to encourage others empowers her further. Sue comes from an alcoholic family and over the years her drinking became more and more habitual. It began with only going out then transpiring into a way of coping emotionally. She recalls the dark time when she felt as though she was a "caged animal" and alcohol became a way in which she found liberation in all the chaos she was enduring. At 19 going through a messy divorce with a child involved and as her Catholic family threatening to disown her due to the divorce, Sue began to consume greater quantities and even attempted suicide.

As things in her life began to improve, the drinking remained constant. She remembers multiple accounts where she would say to herself, "I won't be an alcoholic," however, her drinking began to negatively affect her ability to keep a job and maintain functional relationships. Sue remembers the night at when her husband threatened to take the kids if she didn't get help. Her response continued to be "I am not an alcoholic" but decided to give AA a try. Sue felt she needed more women support and a connection to something greater. AA led Sue to her involvement in Women for Sobriety empowering her to finally finding healing. Sue expressed that the support and involvement with Women for Sobriety gave her the courage to admit to her addiction and stop drinking. What sustained it she expresses was God. She recollects the time that she would blame God and be angry with him. "Why doesn't God stop me?" she would question. One evening it came to her when she was praying "that God doesn't make me drink, but I have to start listening to him. Praying to him and then listening to my heart." Sue began to explore healing modalities such as meditation, spiritual guides, chakra healing, and reiki.

"When my mind starts thinking thoughts like 'what's the use' I retreat to meditation to help bring me back to healthy living. Spiritual healing and holistic treatments were much more effective than the 12 step program. Helping women help women brought me to where I needed to be in order to find healing within. When people ask me how I did it I say all from the help of God."

Sue and many others in life long recovery find sustainable healing from within. Addiction is looking for God in all the wrong places. Many discover abundance and healing when replacing the addiction with something such as spirituality or yoga. Deepak Chopra explains, "Initially our addiction provided us with the rewards we were searching for in our lives; a sense of spiritual well being." It comes from a deep-seated need to belong or feel relief and addiction ranges to food addictions, sex addictions, caffeine, and sugar addictions to behavioral addictions. Healing addiction must first be sourced from within the mind then to rebuild or recondition neurological deficits to heal dysfunctional patterns.

Addictions develop negative patterns within our behavior correlating to the first chakra due to the associated survival and autopilot characteristics. When we provide the body with chemical processes from drugs, for instance, we lose the natural auto-regulation of our innate signaling pathways within the body. Dopamine and endorphins both help produce a sensation of pleasure and ability to deal with pain. These chemical pathways are negatively altered. For example, a single usage of methamphetamine increases our dopamine levels by 1200% and the ability to feel that high again lessens with each subsequent use as the body builds a tolerance to the drug.

This process unfortunately also inhibits one's natural ability to experience joy. In an attempt to achieve the initial high, one spends increasingly excessive amounts of time and money on the addiction, often leading to failed relationships, bankruptcy, and - sometimes - death. This is a pattern that one should avoid at all costs. Whatever the addiction, we should always strive to maintain balance in the body and source that contentment from within- especially since we have the capability to do so.

Furthermore, clinical experience has identified addiction as a growing concern in the U.S. and around the world as well. Though alcohol, tobacco, and drug abuse have occurred for centuries, we now face unprecedented prescription levels - and subsequent addiction - to opioids and other similar medications. In addition to concerns with dependency, there exists the risk for overdosing and potential death caused by these controlled substances. Even the various side effects cause additional medical concerns due to constipation, somnolence, or altered mental status - among other issues.

One of my (KH) most unfortunate experiences involved an unusual case of substance abuse. A 20 year old pregnant female presented to the emergency department in the custody of the local police for altered mental status. She was suspected of polysubstance abuse and had a history of substance abuse. The cachectic patient demonstrated confused thought processes and became combative to the point of pulling out her intravenous therapy lines and her Foley catheter with her feet. Because of this dangerous behavior, drug abuse, and pregnancy - she was admitted to the ICU for close monitoring and medical evaluation.

The patient stated that her drug use increased when her mother was killed 5 months previously. Using the monies awarded from her mother's life insurance policy, the she began purchasing prescription oral narcotics hydroxymorphone and oxymorphone illegally. After several months of standard use, she began crushing and snorting these medications in addition to adding nitrous oxide from aerosol containers.

Because of the chronicity of this addiction and abuse, she experienced bone marrow failure due to substance abuse. Luckily, her bone marrow restarted cell production successfully; however, this negatively affected her pregnancy and postpartum period where her newborn required several weeks of neonatal intensive care for associated complications.

Contemplation, meditation, and solitude are non-drug alternatives to shift perception. Meditation and fasting cultivate releases in the body by directing our thinking to the inner being. Cooking with ghee and coconut oil help heal the digestive tract knowing that proper functioning of the digestive system promotes optimal health. Yoga stimulates neural plasticity, which elevates an addict's ability to heal from the inside out and create new behavioral patterns.

Yoga for Recovery

Yoga empowers the individual, is cost effective, activates mindfulness, benefits all psychological systems, involves Ayurvedic interventions, reduces cortisol, increases heart rate variability, improves breathing, and naturally makes you crave wellbeing. Especially for breaking bad habits, yoga provides a present moment space to yoke the mind, body, and breath tapping into the practitioner's ability to provoke self-healing and self-relaxation.

Another fruitful benefit from practicing yoga is self-study. Because one size does not fit all, the individual must be willing to navigate the essence of body and mind learning what feels right and what doesn't. This can direct the individual into further healing and recovery by cultivating a deeper awareness and presence in each moment to listen to the wisdom of the body and to achieve balance within its systems.

Yoga helps in conjunction with the 12-step program by cultivating awareness of self-destructive behaviors and assisting one with surrendering to a higher power. The 12-step program of Alcoholics Anonymous has exhibited success in helping people stop their addiction setting the foundation to sustain sobriety. However, yoga can help complete the transformation providing tools of mindfulness, breathing techniques, and detoxification furthering recovery to embracing life in its full capacity. Surrender is a prominent component to the 12-steps facilitating acceptance. Admitting powerlessness and unmanageability peels away "denier syndrome" and brings one closer to breaking down ego and realizing that addiction is simply a symptom of underlain issues. Then in stillness of restorative yoga or meditation one can feel infused with positive affirmations of "I am okay, in this present moment." From there a new lens on facing the underlain issues can illuminate truth and pave a path to sustainable healing.

Restoring back to sanity begins with surrender and attending the present moment as it is. Yoga is a tool to come home to yourself and instills self-acceptance as a by product of present moment awareness. We often categorize love with another being and in addiction love becomes associated with "it." But beginning to cultivate a deeper connection and an openness to love, we begin to realize that love exists now. We hold an organic capacity to hold ourselves with love and we do not need to be loved back. We love to love and by self-care practices generating self-love grounds us back into balance. Turning off the controlling mind, and turning on a deep connection within. By opening that connection it creates a deeper capacity to listen and to be restored.

Addiction is a compulsion to control multiple elements in one's life. Step number three is the definition of surrender, "Made a decision to turn our will and our lives over to the care of God as we understood Him." The balance of letting go but keeping faith. This is surrender. It is choosing to give the power over in relief knowing you do not have all the answers and the bigger picture is in someone else's hands. And the yoga practice enhances our approach to God by living moment-by-moment, breath-by-breath. Bhakti yoga is the yoga of devotional love, which offers a way to grow closer in gratitude to the healing experiences of surrendering.

> **"I avoid looking forward or backward,**
> **and try to keep looking upward."**
> **–Charlotte Bronte**

Creating a fearless moral inventory of ourselves exemplifies self-study, which is a key practice in the eight limbs of yoga. Searching and taking a fearless moral inventory of ourselves requires courage and humility to see the right path. In yoga, Tapas means burning up impurities by practice. It is the detoxifying element yoga has to offer- acknowledging challenge, illusion, or illness and releasing it through the body. Adopting a practice that supports the cleansing process on a deeper level paves the way to consciously derail emotional disturbances that may initiate relapse or counterproductive thoughts. Tapas meaning "heat" in Sanskrit and is used as a verb meaning "to hurt," or "to cause pain." Ancient yogis noted that the elements of the earth are also within our bodies. They noticed it was through fire that purification happened, thus gold is purified through fire. This idea of burning one's 'impurities' is essentially a formula to release dysfunctional patterns. Swami Kripalu describes tapas as doing something you wouldn't normally do, or simply stepping outside of your comfort zone. In the yoga practice, tapas are exemplified through the practitioner's discipline. For example, if a strengthening pose is very challenging by taking another breath or holding it for one more moment- that is practicing tapas. It is a cleansing way to transform one into a deeper capacity to hold. The discipline itself cultivates our ability to create space between our thoughts and our emotions- so not identifying completely with something that might possibly change like "I am weak," "I cannot do this," or other negative associations of who we are. Instead, thoughts such as "This is temporary, each moment is temporary," "I am enough," "I am brave," and "I am strong." The discipline creates space between our emotions and our reactions yielding fruits of patience, self-reflection, and understanding thus creating an opportunity to pause and consider before making a destructive decision.

The Yoga practice if summed up teaches resilience in change. We show up on the mat or in the moment having no prerequisites to qualify us worthy of practicing. There is no particular belief system necessary and no level of fitness or flexibility necessary. We show up willing to surrender and witness the experience generating a type of change. Changes such as, removing thoughts or illness, bringing unity within the mind and body, or redirecting our thought patterns to the present moment begin to instill a different type of freedom within us- a freedom that no one but ourselves has permission to take away.

With community support and recreating new thought platforms to encourage one self, the individual can detoxify the physical body from patterns or substance and renew the mind with discipline. The practice of yoga, breath work, and meditation naturally releases the impurities, or tapas, and harvests a lot of potential in supporting the progress for someone who is on the road to recovery.

Step five is the process of acknowledging and correlates with the fifth chakra component of this book. A way to get honest with yourself is by witnessing your thoughts during meditation. Noticing what arises, but do not become attached. Practice being present with yourself. To heal others, we must begin with healing ourselves first. Step six expresses the alchemy that takes place in yoga the moment we begin the practice playing a key role in surrender. It is the perception that carries one from challenging poses to relaxation and encourages our ability to detach from the negative, false identities we may place on ourselves. Letting go of what doesn't serve you, to create space for what does moving into the seventh step of 'humbly asking Him to remove our shortcomings'. It is important to meet yourself where you are at all times. As self-awareness is heightened through yoga and meditation; prayer is a heartfelt communication that enables us to surrender and release our fears. Life is a fluctuating journey and the moment we discharge the perception of perfection but begin with what is in this moment, then growth can manifest. Furthermore, the ability to let go of identifying yourself as broken or as an addict, but embracing that these are simply challenges intended to refine you- if you allow it to.

Mantra: "I am not my challenges or circumstances. I am whole. I am open to the unlimited possibilities of growth and strive to be a better version of myself each day."

The eighth and ninth steps are really all about taking the steps necessary towards making amends and healing by cultivating the courage to move through your fears and into love. This is a prime example of taking what you do off the mat and into the world. Adopting non-harming (ahimsa) is one of the five yamas within the eight limbs of yoga which creates a solid foundation to peace. As you are more clear on what you need during the process of healing, be sure to create the patience and space necessary to maintain non-violence. Yoga is an ever-evolving adventure seeped into self awareness and care. By creating an intention of witnessing your personal inventory during your practice, it may help clarify what you need to keep improving and progress. As one practices witnessing and tuning in, the tenth step about continuing to take personal inventory and accountability becomes more and more natural in redesigning relationships, trust, and wellness.

The eleventh step regarding seeking through prayer and meditation to improve our conscious contact with God, as we understood Him, praying only for knowledge of His will for us and the power to carry that out is a foundation in seventh chakra balance and living out what we are meant to. I often teach that yoga practice is a way of coming home to yourself where prayer and meditation is a way of coming home to God. Yoga has a way of disciplining the mind and body by rather than reacting we respond, rather than believing emotional disturbances we witness. When the mind begins to heal the body will follow. Step twelve is a psycho-social step in which we carry the discipline and lessons learned from our healing off the yoga mat and into our lives. It's no longer passing hurt on but expanding deeper into our wholeness of who we are beneath the stories. A sober, clear mind is expansive empowering one in all the quadrants of life.

Whether sourced from therapeutic interventions, the Twelve Steps, faith, a mind-body approach - or all the above - the acknowledgement of spiritual well being has shown to play a significant role in helping people break the cycle of addiction. By uncovering the underlying causes of imbalances addiction can be alleviated, but the mental, physical, and spiritual components of health must be addressed. As we live in a culture of desire, Carl Jung who founded analytical psychology suggests that addiction is an illness only spirituality can heal. Creating treatments from the spirit allows one to connect to a deeper meaning of life identifying all obstacles as an opportunity for growth grounding back into his or her journey of growth and potential.

Eating Disorders

In early work with treating eating disorders, the assumption was that eating disorders stem from a desire to acquire a locust of control in one's life. As that may hold true in some cases, a chakra perspective may identify eating disorders as coming from an underlying imbalance of being unrooted. Essentially, eating disorders can reflect an imbalance in the root chakra. Food was designed to sustain our bodies. From the beginning of time, humans have utilized food as nourishment and medication. Using sustenance as a form of abuse can symbolize separation of mind from body and be exemplified by overeating to create a sense of security or even starving oneself due to feeling inadequate. The right to live or to be is an imperative aspect of a balanced root chakra; thus, when we deny our source of nourishment or obsessing over being thin, one must evaluate his or her feelings involving security and the right to live.

Obsessing over food can be a way one feels the right to choose and when there is an imbalance in the root chakra, one can become consumed with dysfunctional eating habits by becoming attached to numbers (calories, scale, etc.) and even honing into saying no to eating. This is especially apparent for someone who feels a lack of power or authority over his or her life. Furthermore, this false sense of security grants the individual with the perceived power of controlling his or her physical appearance.

On the other end of the spectrum, overeating that leads to weight gain can stem from feeling inadequate, insecure, shame, and/or repressed emotion. Body fat is used as insulation to regulate our temperature protecting us from extreme cold or heat. When one feels insecure or shame regarding their right to live or threatened by social and environmental conditions, the body will begin to insulate creating layers to protect. This unhealthy sense of security leads to many other health imbalances such as diabetes, heart problems, and high blood pressure.

Each component can benefit by grounding into a sustainable relationship with the body and returning to the foundation of nourishment. As the first chakra relates with survival, security, and potential; creating a safe space to start self care practices such as self massage, yoga, and mindfulness can begin to ground the individual back to feeling safe in the body. From there focusing on affirmation and growth by reconstructing personal identity with the present moment begins to pave a path leading to higher potential and wellness.

David McClelland developed the acquired needs theory which proposes that every person holds an aspiration for achievement, power, and affiliation. Each can be attained by a balanced root chakra. When one becomes devoted to personal development through physical, mental, and spiritual growth, this provides a sense of meaning for the individual. In addition, power is accomplished simply in our right to exist and how our presence contributes and influences different factors within our life. From birth, we may experience affiliation with family or care givers. When this need isn't met over time, it can manifest into mental and physical maladies. It is human nature to affiliate with someone or something- regardless of the companionship or relationship- feeling supported by another being cultivates a sense of security due to the fact that we as humans are naturally social and have thrived based off of connection and community since the beginning of time.

Self Healing Tools

View Yoga Glossary for First Chakra Yoga Poses

Foot Massage-
Our feet literally carry us through each day. Massaging them each morning, focusing on the soles in particular, is a very grounding

and nurturing practice. But because various points on the feet correlate with organs and tissues throughout the body, it also supports proper vision, relieves stress, and offers many other systemic benefits. This in conjunction with wiggling the toes, or feeling your feet planting into the ground (earthing) also supports shifting the first chakra into balance.

Walking Meditation (pg. 113)

Mindful Practices

Yoga Nidra (pg. 125)

The Yamas

The yamas, one of the eight limbs of yoga, serve as restraints that you put on yourself to decrease the suffering of another being. The yamas include non-harming, truthfulness, non-stealing, non-greed, and moderation. Practicing these concepts help bring balance into our lives by cultivating peace and also prevents us from feeling drained by things that are dysfunctional and unsustainable. By fortifying these character traits it helps reduce suffering within our lives, within ourselves, and our relationship with others.

Our attitude and behavior essentially construct the reality in which we live. Practicing non-harming invites us to create space between our thoughts and actions to witness the consequences and repercussions of reactive behavior. Often time, harming is not just physically hurting someone- but is derived from fear. In our fear, we become clouded so we may use our words in attempt to punish others or manipulate with selfish intent. Non-harming is not dependent on others, but is manifested from our relationship with ourselves. Are you participating in self sabotage, self neglect, or illusion? If we are harming others, often it is a reflection of self abuse and sabotage. The first step in redirecting behavior is witnessing it. We must be mindful in order to change.

It takes more energy to pull oneself out of a lie than to simply tell the truth. Lying includes and is not limited to; manipulating truth, justifying harm, withholding holding authentic feelings, and neglecting what is real. Honesty is sustainable and requires integrity to our lives, self and others. When we compromise truth, we become unrooted and deprived of authenticity. Eventually, if we continue to reject truth, the winds of deceit will rip trust and peace away. It takes courage to be honest, however, when we sit back taking inquiry of the costs of being dishonest- one must consider the weight. Consider how when one falls into the pattern lying, his or her reality shifts into the maintenance of distortion creating a path leading one away from who they truly are. Although truth is manifested at the fifth chakra, when truth is distorted, it debilitates the root chakra throwing everything else off balance.

So often, we steal from others without even realizing it. Entitlement is one of the must under-acknowledged forms of stealing. It is derived from attachment and the fear of lack cultivating a storm of selfishness and karmic imbalance. In order to receive we must share an offering. When we assume we are automatically permitted to emotional, physical, or material things- we begin to create expectation which will always result in disappointment and inadequacy. The mindset alone has the potential to wreck possibilities and interrupt entelechial development. Stealing is lying and harming. Even if we are not deliberately taking an object from someone- but even through trying to be a carbon copy of something or recycling the intellectual property of another claiming it to be yours is stealing. We steal experiences from those we love through the justification of 'busyness'. We steal time from people blinded by our perceived needs or lack of accountability. We even steal educational and experiential learning opportunities from others through inserting unsolicited counsel. Stealing takes many shapes, be mindful of the ways stealing takes shape in your life.

Non-greed is the continued practice of letting go of what does not serve. It is the deep understanding that nothing actually belongs to us in this life and everything is temporary. There is peace and contentment in the simple through non-attachment. Non-attachment liberates us from fear based illusions allowing us to truly enjoy the details of living and loving. When we try to possess and control the things within our lives, one often becomes let down due to the attachment of an expectation or over identifying with something. Furthermore, trying to possess and control often impacts and harms another human. We may be attempting to direct another's path in the way we assume they should go, or pressuring someone to be something they are not. Many years become wasted through this chasing and trying to possess a vision, a person, a want, an exception- where as if we begin to release the feeling of neediness, contentment surfaces. Letting go is the purest form of liberation.

Moderation is wrapped in contentment and gratitude. It is illustrated in simplicity and non-hoarding. Excessiveness is fear and longing. We must be mindful in our over indulgences acknowledging where the false sense of security is coming from. When we are treading in a pool of excess, we must begin to strip away the layers to tune into what we really need. It is not about deprivation, but honoring what we truly need in the present moment with containment and self control. As we reconnect with ourselves, taking inquiry of the whispers within we can explore; is it loneliness? Boredom? Fear? Inadequacy? The longings that cry deep within us that often cause the desire for excess is really a longing to be connected with God. It is through our body and the act of tuning into meditation, nourishing ourselves through movement and healthy eating- that we can begin to fill that longing. The moment we realize we already have everything we need, this imbalance dissipates. It takes knowing this at a cellular level, that we are supported and have the right to live and everything we already need; we can source our own peace rather than attempting to extract it from external things. Tune into humility, shed the layers, come home to yourself.

By adopting these characteristics, one becomes connected at the heart of who they are staying rooted in peace. These five principles lay a solid foundation to invite peace and sustainability into life. The yamas serve as preventative health and education as those who live aligned to these have less stress and higher resilience. Often times, to correct imbalance, one can redirect cognitive perceptions and reorganize a life into wellness. No doctor, therapist, friend, or teacher can force another to live in balance- the individual must take accountability to reflect and redirect to achieve balance, wholeness, and peace.

Grounding Breath Visualization

Sitting comfortably, begin to close your eyes. Take a deep breath in through the nose feeling the breath rise from the base of your spine into your forehead. On your exhale, imagine the breath flowing down the body into the pelvic floor rooting. On the inhale draw that energy from the pelvic floor feeling it rise up into the forehead and again slowly exhale feeling the breath travel down into the earth. Every breath, feel the breath rooting deeper into the ground below your pelvic floor- and the inhales drawing nutrients from that. Rooting down with the exhale to rise up with the inhale. Imagine every exhale digging deeper into the earth, maybe feeling as though the exhale is growing roots into the ground. Every inhale infuses the body with more nourishment and every exhale your roots grow deeper into the earth. Continue this for as long as you like. Grounding yourself into this moment. For your breath is the vehicle to now.

SACRAL CHAKRA

Wellness is Movement

~~~

Trust only movement. Life happens at the level of events, not of words. Trust movement. -Alfred Adler

The sacral chakra is the second of the chakras located in the lumbar sacral plexus and the organs associated are the womb, genitals, bladder, and kidneys. The glands associated with this chakra are the ovaries, which secrete both estrogen and progesterone, and the testes, which produce testosterone. Svadhishthana is the Sanskrit word for the second chakra meaning, "in one's own abode." In the chakra story this is the space where mundane life is interrupted by stress, trauma, or suffering. When one experiences trauma in his or her life, the body stores the trauma and eventually it begins to surface through behavior and illness if not faced or dealt with. Trauma must be integrated through the body. The element here is water representing the idea that we went from a solid foundation to the water where feelings of uncertainty, shock, and transformation may occur.

The sacral chakra is a 'make or break you' space opening the opportunity for rebirth or awakening. The fluidity element reflects our ability to be resilient and flow like water. This can be observed through the mantra, "life happens through me, not to me." The shadow here holds guilt and the victim archetype, but can be countered through harnessing the right to feel and moving through the disturbance sourcing courage to tap into self care and power to keep 'flowing'. A crescent moon is the symbol indicating the light in darkness, victory over death, rebirth, and exposing what is false by illuminating truth. Imbalances reflect indifference, neglect, belittlement to others, stupor, indulgences like substance abuse and addiction, distrust, cruelty, helplessness, and loss of common sense. The color is moonlight on water with the idea that one heals when he or she makes sense or acceptance of suffering. Meaning must be made for transformation to occur.

The second chakra's other attributes include procreation, sense of taste, sense organ is tongue, work organs are the genitals, fantasy, attention to desires that fulfill sensory enjoyment, an interest in art, music, and poetry, personal archetypes begin to develop, and sexuality. There is a psychological correlation with movement and connection, which help balance the second chakra. However, the negative mind can easily take control instilling feelings of emptiness and purposelessness when adversity, restrictions, and unwanted discipline appear in one's life making it crucial that balancing and self-care are obtained to remain well. Later in the chapter there will be balancing techniques to support one in coping in these challenges.

A Medical Lens

Modern medicine can medically account for several of the pathologies associated with this chakra because of their physical locations in relation to the chakra. Due to the proximity to the root chakra, many of the same internal organs - and subsequent health issues - overlap. This is seen in multiple areas from sexual dysfunction to bladder problems like bed-wetting. Reproductive health in men and women - with potential problems including endometriosis, infertility, testicular or prostate disease, and dysmenorrhea - take place here. Like the root chakra, the GI system is also co-located here, hence many GI pathologies. This is why the presence of stress, trauma, or suffering can precipitate episodes of bowel pathologies like IBS or Crohn's Disease, which can also be attributed to the sacral chakra.

Furthermore, there are many neurological connections to the various nearby organ systems and distant parts of the body that can cause pain or dysfunction. Any localized nerve trauma, compression, or infection may attribute to these maladies. Specifically, the sacral plexus contributes to various sensory and motor functions of the legs, pelvis, and buttocks. Any malfunction may cause a subsequent decrease in function at the associated location.

Yoga and Trauma Recovery

Military

During the September 2014 American Veteran and Community Center Advisory Committee meeting, Captain Ivan Castro shared his story to the group. He began with explaining how most soldiers see deployments in black and white. White being they come home alive and black being they come home in a coffin. However, soldiers often do not prepare for the grey area in between. The long term sequelae encompasses anything from missing limbs to the invisible injuries such as PTSD. PTSD (Post Traumatic Stress Disorder) and TBI (Traumatic Brain Injury) are two of the most common and challenging conditions soldiers return from war with cultivating symptoms causing it to be an even deeper challenge to reintegrate back into civilian life. More than two million service members have deployed in support of operations in Afghanistan and Iraq since the terrorist attacks on September 11th 2001. As the Veterans Health Administration has spent billions of dollars to treat veterans of recent overseas contingency operations, the costs are only rising in combating these "grey area" wounds.

The current treatment and rehabilitation methods statistically have been failing our service members from pain medication addictions to suicide rates, therefore, implementing new modalities supported by evidence based research may have a remarkable result in healing PTSD and TBI. When you couple somatic practices with cognitive processing, healing occurs on an astounding level.

TBI

Traumatic Brain Injury, also known as TBI, is caused by trauma to the head and is represented through a broad range of symptoms such as decreased level of consciousness, amnesia, or neurological abnormalities. Soldiers who have been exposed to explosions or any blunt force trauma to the head commonly are diagnosed with TBI. Because of the complexity of the brain and the variability of symptom presentation, finding appropriate treatment for the individual has been a trying problem for the VA. Millions of Americans have TBI and the injuries are not only difficult to live with, but also very expensive to treat. Even with treatment, there has been no actual cure; however, one way to alleviate the ailments of TBI can be demonstrated through yoga practice. The world of TBI and yoga is a newly touched subject where there are not many studies out there, however, many soldiers who have participated in classes report improved sleep, less pain, and a better outlook on life. I had the privilege of seeing first hand the effects of yoga for TBI.

As I was teaching a mindfulness and yoga workshop to wounded warriors from The Wounded Warrior Project, we were discussing hope through lifestyle choice, one veteran had the courage to speak of his story and opinion on healing TBI. He expressed his frustration of having to see many therapists, being prescribed many medications, and seeing no results. With teary eyes and a dour tone, he told me that his doctor at the VA told him there was no hope in him healing. That he is broken and will simply have to live with it. However, he disagreed because since he began taking my classes and workshops he began to see a difference in the way he felt, the quality of sleep, and his ability to control his anger. By the end of our series together he shared his testimony to the practice. He explained that because of his improvements he was able to decrease the dosage of his medications and found that because of meditation and yoga nidra he was sleeping through the night and was less reactive throughout the day. His wife disclosed with me that his demeanor is so different since he began practicing and how imperative these modalities are for TBI and PTSD. Over my time working with veterans and the military demographic, these testimonies are very common instilling more hope for many to find healing to their injury.

PTSD

Post Traumatic Stress Disorder is a type of anxiety disorder that is bred from a traumatic experience. It is a normal reaction to an abnormal situation that devastates the person's ability to adapt or cope with life. Trauma comes from the Greek word meaning "wound." It essentially separates the mind from the body causing hyper-arousal, anxiety, depression, addiction, and other maladies in the mind and body. As trauma notoriously separates the body from the mind, healing must begin within the body.

Addressing Second Chakra and the Psoas Muscle

The Psoas Major is a fusiform muscle located on the side of the lumbar region of the vertebral column that extends through the lesser pelvis area. It connects the iliacus muscle to iliopsoas, meaning it runs through the front of the low back through the pelvis to the top of the leg. It resides deep within the pelvis contributing to flexion of the hip joint function to pull the leg towards the body when the body is fixed or pulls the body towards the leg when the leg is fixed.

The Psoas, however, is much more than a muscle. It performs neurological behavior in relationship to trauma. The autonomic part of the nervous system will activate the psoas in response to a threat. This is part of the sympathetic nervous system's fight or flight response. When the nervous system is under constant hyper arousal as a result from anxiety disorders such as PTSD, the psoas becomes over activated and does not relax properly.

For instance, when we hear a loud crash the body reflexively ducks down- this is the psoas being activated. An over activated psoas becomes weak and sends signals of disorganization back to the brain. When there is proper balance between the body and nervous system, the psoas participates in proprioception, which is our perception of our body in space. In other words, proprioception is an approach to how we feel safe in our body. A hyperactive psoas keeps the brain-body continuum in a constant state of alert. The parasympathetic nervous system deactivates the sympathetic nervous system and the body/hormone reactions to bring one back into a natural state of wellbeing. But if there is not a balance between the parasympathetic nervous system and sympathetic nervous system, the body cannot return back to its natural state of functioning.

Imagine a water faucet with hot water being sympathetic nervous system (fight and flight) and cold water being the parasympathetic nervous system (rest and digest). In order for the water to not burn you when you turn the hot water on you turn cold water on the balance it out into a comfortable temperature. If one is under a constant state of fight or flight it and there is no rest and digest to balance it out; the body cannot find a comfortable balance causing disorganization and eventually illness. However, if we activate the parasympathetic nervous system- so as to turn cold water on- we can become more resilient to stress (the scorching hot water). But in order for there to be balance, one must practice ways of resilience and relaxation to stimulate the parasympathetic nervous system - to cool the nervous system.

The same autonomic stimulation for rest and digest also allows signals our body to repair and heal. This is a moment of self-maintenance and care for the body - something that cannot occur effectively in a state of constant arousal. A weak, abused psoas often can lead to chronic pain within the pelvis region, neck and shoulder pain, or other illnesses. The psoas is not a muscle to work out or stretch to repair but to utilize stress resilience in order to heal a hyper-aroused nervous system. The idea is that resolving what caused the hyperarousal will heal the abused psoas.

Healing

There is no question that psychology has significantly influenced our understanding of the psyche itself; however, as we advance in science and understanding the effects of trauma, the approaches to healing remain limited. Neurology explores more in depth about how the brain processes life experiences, thus, leading to a deeper potential of healing not only within the mind but the whole organism. Often times when one is seeking resolution from trauma the first response is go see a psychologist and talk about the story.

However, the body itself does not communicate verbally - rather the body communicates via sensation and, therefore, may need to employ healing methods beyond traditional psychological clinical visits. Many patients have difficulties recalling traumatic events due to protective mechanisms of the body. The organism does not care about the story, rather protecting the individual so he or she may best survive the event. Often times, the musculoskeletal and nervous systems will store tension through muscle memory or neural networks - supporting the argument that healing must come from a somatic release. The restructuring of neural patterns does not even need to talk about the story or relive the experience; but through building resilience in the nervous system, coming out of an opioid response, or activating neural plasticity. All of these benefits may be achieved through meditation practices, self massage, and yoga.

Why Yoga Heals

Yoga means "to yoke" the mind, body, and spirit. While trauma disrupts the baseline mechanisms within the body, yoga encompasses techniques to counter or heal such disruption and bring harmony back into the mind and body. Often times cognitive therapies are used to support soldiers and veterans who face PTSD, but these cognitive therapies can only go so far because the body has stored the trauma into the nervous system, limbic brain, and muscle memory. With this in mind, somatic practices like yoga are wonderful ways to release stored tension and trauma from the body.

Yoga has the capacity to expand our ability for self understanding above and beyond the wounds and past experiences. A Texas veteran said, "yoga shows me what is right with me." Many healing modalities in conventional medicine repeatedly remind the patient what is wrong with their mind or body, whereas yoga teaches that your identity is not your wounds, not your challenges, and not your mistakes. This mindfulness practice supports the individual in reconstructing their reality and regaining control during everyday life.

Beginning with the mind, yoga supports healing on many levels. Neural plasticity describes the brain's capacity to change neural connectivity and pathways in response to new experiences. For example, in yoga practice the use of meditation and intention allow veterans to develop a new lens in their relationship with themselves. Whether using breathing to control the way they feel in a challenging pose or to stimulate their own relaxation, the individual begins to source his or her own peace allowing for repair of the hyper aroused nervous system and associated anxiety. Also, the use of new pleasurable neuromuscular pathways (movement patterns) derails painful neural signals helping the body release tension and/or pain. Great yoga practices for this specifically are yoga nidra (integrative restoration), meditative flow, and meditation.

Furthermore, different poses or stretches have an impact on the endocrine system, which stimulates the secretion and production of hormones in the body. As an added benefit, the poses themselves render empowerment, strength, flexibility, and holistic healing in the body's muscles, posture, and breath capacity. Through the implementation of breath and movement, the nervous system begins to balance between the "fight or flight" and the "rest and digest" building stress resilience. Yoga conditions resilience through demanding physical poses while teaching the one to soften and relax using breath and patience to exemplify how temporary the challenge is. Many principles can be taken off the yoga mat and into the one's life, such as transforming his or her pain into wisdom and challenges into assignments to grow. This empowerment creates new thinking patterns to support acceptance and healing in the mind.

The body has an innate ability to heal itself. When one couples somatic practices with cognitive processes, healing occurs on an astounding level. Author of "Odysseus in America," Dr. Jonathan Shay expresses that post traumatic stress disorder should be renamed post traumatic stress injury because this is not a permanent disorder, veterans can be cured and experience a happy full life after war. Our veterans and soldiers deserve to live in the freedom that they are fighting for. With further implementation of yoga therapy for those suffering from the "grey area" of post deployment life, there will be continued hope in re-gaining inner peace and wellness in each quadrants of his or her health.

Yoga

Yoga practice has the capacity to expand our knowing of who we are outside of our experiences. The practice has a remarkable way of directing the practitioner's focus into the present moment unshackling him or her from their "wounded," "broken" identity. Unfortunately, often times when one experiences trauma they begin to self identify with the experience or their inability to get past that experience. When one takes a full hour away from the false identity and into acceptance of what the present moment brings, it extends their perspective only to the openness of what is now- not what happened a few hours ago, days ago, years ago- or who they fear they will be in the future. By bringing the mind into the present moment it begins the mend proprioception and self-identity. Proprioception in short, is the ability to feel safe in one's body. It is how we perceive our body in space relative to our position of neighboring parts within the body and how we employ movement. Through self-massage and fluid body movements, one can improve proprioception by mind body integration. And through adding breath into the movements it improves heart rate variability, increases parasympathetic responses within the nervous system, and brings ease into the mind through concentration of the present moment. Furthermore, this begins to instill new pleasurable neuromuscular pathways to derail painful pathways within the body.

Using yoga poses, breathing practices, and meditation to tolerate and access the trauma stored in the body builds resilience and the ability to heal from the inside out. This is not an overnight treatment but a lifestyle change that heals the wound rather than silencing the symptoms. Be patient with this sustainable healing because this is you healing you. Practice makes permanence. Yoga facilitates the alchemy of transforming pain into wisdom. So using affirmations and knowing that the challenge is simply an assignment to grow.

Self Healing Tools

For facing PTSD or other anxiety disorders the most efficient, holistic way of healing is through quiet intuitive practices such as meditation (page), meditative flow yoga, breathing practices, and prayer.

Mindful Practice

Yoga Nidra (pg. 125)

Grounding and Self Care

The most imperative aspect to healing is having a proper understanding and insight into one's current state. Honoring each limitation you face through acceptance opens the capacity to change it. As Rumi once said, "The cure for pain is in the pain." Reminding us that we must meet it to get through it. In life, we must accept that pain is inevitable; however, suffering is optional. By taking steps to connect with ways of self care to elevate our potential of healing, use the tools around you to manage it. Whether it be sharing compassion with someone who has experienced something similar as you or journaling the authentic way you feel. Finding ways to establish safety cultivates recovery. As Judith Herman discusses in her book Trauma and Recovery "it should be possible to recognize a gradual shift from unpredictable danger to reliable safety, from dissociated trauma to acknowledged memory, and from stigmatized isolation to restored social connect." (p. 155) To establish this safety one must be willing to focus on gaining control within the body- as yoga, meditation, and self care guide one into that space- then moving outside the body into control of the environment.

"The most important decision we make is whether we believe we live in a friendly or a hostile universe." –Albert Einstein

Whether practicing journaling or meditation, we empower ourselves to choose who and what has permission to wound us, creating an opportunity to orchestrate our future in the way in which we desire. If being somewhere exhausts you or makes you uncomfortable, give yourself permission to say "no." This honors yourself and your healing. If being alone for the afternoon is what you need, then take that time to be with yourself. These simple choices constructs one's aptitude for self care.

A poem called Letting Go, author unknown, sheds light into what it really means to let go. Utilizing these statements or mantras as affirmation within the process of letting go, can derive personal empowerment, self actualization, and deep rooted healing. Below are segments from the poem.

To "let go" does not mean to stop caring;
it means I can't do it for someone else.

To "let go" is not to enable,
but to allow learning from natural consequences.

To "let go" is to admit powerlessness;
which means the outcome is not in my hands.

To "let go" is not to fix,
but to be supportive.

To "let go" is not to deny,
but to accept.

To "let go" is not to adjust everything to my desires
but to take each day as it comes,
and cherish myself in it.

To "let go" is not to regret the past,
but to grow and live for the future.

To "let go" is to fear less,
and love more.

Body

View Yoga Glossary for Second Chakra Yoga Poses

Neurogenic Tremor

Imagine an image of the African plains. A group of gazelles suddenly sees a lion coming from the bushes to attack one of the gazelles and kills it. How is it that the gazelles can go from such a traumatic experience in nature - witnessing one of their family eaten by a lion - and then five minutes later be calmly drinking from the water hole? Ingrained in the mammal's nervous system is an innate way of discharging excessive tension through rapid muscle contraction and relaxation to calm the body down from a hyper-aroused adrenal state. Mammals will shake forcefully, allowing the nervous system to release the trauma. Likewise, we as mammals have the same functioning within our bodies. In situations of traumatic stress (like after being in a car accident), or physical stress (like after childbirth) you may feel your body begin to shake or even if you are really upset the body may begin to shake - this is called neurogenic shaking.

In our culture however, we are often told to stop shaking or we try to suppress the shaking within our bodies - cutting off the organism's natural way of processing the trauma as result leading to dysfunctions such as chronic pain or muscle tension rather than the body being brought back into balance. As recent studies have brought attention to the healing effects of neurogenic trembling, the shaking creates a vibration of contraction and ease that releases the built up tension held in the muscles and connective tissue of the body stimulating the parasympathetic nervous system. The brainstem initiates a discharge of the physical tension associated with the event. During neurogenic shaking practices, one does not have to think of the event but simply just be in the body. It goes back to the body communication via sensation rather than verbal language. These exercises are used to induce the tremors from the psoas then evoking the other muscles throughout the body. One may combine yoga poses and breathing exercises with neurogenic shaking re-awaking the body's intrinsic release mechanism for healing an embedded trauma.

The idea is to use strengthening poses from yoga to fatigue the leg muscles. You may even experience neurogenic shaking from sitting at the edge of your seat and gently lifting your heel letting the muscles relax and thus the leg may tremor. In David Berceli's book *The Revolutionary Trauma Release Process,* he not only provides wonderful information about neurology and how the body is affected by trauma but he teaches many exercises for neurogenic shaking within his program The Trauma Release Process.

So whether you feel the pulses inside the body causing you to shake or you randomly begin to shake - let it be. Neurogenic shaking allows the body to process built up tension stored from hyper arousal, thus, flushing it out.

Breath Work

Alternate Nostril Breathing

Seated in a comfortable position lift the right hand bringing up your index finger and middle finger- like a peace sign. Drop the index and middle finger lifting the thumb, ring, and pinky fingers. Bring your hand to the front of your nose. Take a deep breath in through both nostrils. When you begin to exhale press your thumb against the right nostril. Once the exhale is complete inhale back in through the left nostril. Close the left nostril with your ring finger and exhale out the right nostril. Inhale back through the right nostril closing the right nostril and exhale out the left nostril. Inhale back through the left nostril, closing the left nostril, exhale out the right. Continue this for three to five minutes.

Once you are finished lower your hand down and inhale deeply through both nostrils and then sigh it out. Take a moment and pause after exhaling to witness how the body feels, the face, the hands. Practicing this awareness helps one soften and carry that relaxation with them after they've practiced alternative nostril breathing.

This breathing practice is a great way to refresh the mind as it instills clarity and improves brain functioning. Because alternative nostril breathing infuses the body with equal amounts of oxygen to both sides of the brain it improves our ability to use both sides of the brain with more concentration and accuracy. Alternative Nostril Breathing merges the thinking brain (left) and feeling brain (right) while encouraging a calmer emotional state, regulating the cooling and warming cycles of the body, soothes the nervous system, and improves ability to sleep. It is also a great way to begin a meditation practice.

The Anti-Anxiety Breath

Something to note about breathing is that long exhale activate parasympathetic functioning in the nervous system. The act of inhalation activates the body; therefore, when facing PTSD or any type of anxiety disorder one must focus on prolonged exhales which are a great way to calm the body and improve sleep.

Begin by sitting in a position where the spine can remain comfortably upright. Focus your attention inward noticing how your natural breath feels in the body. Breathing in through the nose and out the nose. On your next exhalation release the air from the nostrils slower than while inhaling. After the exhale hold the breath out for three counts (approximately 3 seconds). Inhale again slowly through the nose, then exhale as slowly as possible out the nose- hold. Inhale slowly, exhale even slower and hold. Repeat this for ten rounds.

Implementing affirmations - such as those listed below - to the breathing are very helpful to directing focus.

"I am calm and peaceful in the now" (Inhale)
"I release all my anxieties" (Exhale)
"I accept all present moments" (Inhale)
"I release concerns" (Exhale)
"I enjoy life" (Inhale)
"I am peaceful" (Exhale)

SOLAR PLEXUS CHAKRA

Sourcing Your Power

~~~~~

"The most common way people give up their power is by thinking they don't have any." ~ Alice Walker

The third chakra is located at the solar plexus within the navel region. The glands and hormones related to this chakra are adrenals, pancreas, liver, stomach, duodenum, kidneys, and adipose tissue. Manipura is the Sanskrit name meaning 'the city of jewels' as this is where we mine our energy making it the power center of the body. This is the space of alchemy holding great physical and energetic wealth. The element of the third chakra is fire. Furthermore, this is where we process personal transformation alchemizing our suffering into wisdom, transforming our desires into goals, and digesting our experiences into lessons. For alchemy to occur there must be an application of heat and pressure making this the source of our motivation as well as where our energetic deficiencies come from. Since this is the location where the body converts food to energy literally a degree of digestion or alchemy needs to occur in order for one to be well.

Characteristics include the color 'embers of fire', self-actualization, sensory of sight, "I will," too much ego, personal power, and improvement. When the third chakra is balanced it is easier for one to access energy and motivation within his or her life. When the desires manifested from the previous chakras (1st and 2nd) become domesticated balance ensues. However, when trauma or stress have not been met, then imbalances including timidity, shame, fear, envy, sadistic behaviors, neurosis, lethargy, depression, disempowerment, unhealthy competition, suppressed emotion, denial, yearning for power, infatuation, and hatred begin to surface. This chakra exhibits a place of intense emotion and is associated with the "gut brain."

Some call this the gut feeling, which is attributed to one's enteric nervous system. The sensitivity of the 100 million neurons (which is more neurons than in the parasympathetic nervous system) exist in this emotional center. 90 percent of fibers in the vagus nerve carry information from the body to the brain activating the limbic system as a way of comforting the brain. For example, when one is faced with extreme stress or anxiety that triggers the limbic system, the vagus nerve carries information back to the brain that activates a fight/flight response or the opposite- a rest and digest response. Furthermore, just like the brain, there are over thirty neurotransmitters located here. The gut brain is a highly sensitive place and studies are now indicating that emotional wellbeing not only takes place in the brain above but also in the brain below.

Gut Brain

Our digestive system is very complex and is as imperative as the mind itself. Our thinking brain generates our ability to comprehend and integrate experiences with wisdom, understanding, and our inner world. The thinking brain sources our decision-making and behavior. The gut brain, however, facilitates digestion and defense.

It senses digestive discomfort and feelings playing key roles in certain diseases accumulated throughout the body. There is no conscious thoughts or choice making, yet the gut brain consists of sheaths of neurons embedded in the alimentary canal. Like the thinking brain, the gut brain has over thirty neurotransmitters and consists of 100 million neurons, which is more than both the spinal cord or the peripheral nervous system.

Michael Gershon, author of The Second Brain, talks about the interesting correlation between depression treatments and side effects. Furthermore, he explains that many therapist uses electrical stimulation of the vagus nerve targeting the mind to treat depression, which may unintentionally impact the gut. In fact, 95 percent of the body's serotonin is found within the bowels. Because antidepressant medications called selective serotonin reuptake inhibitors increase serotonin levels, it's little wonder that meds meant to cause chemical changes in the mind often provoke GI issues such as IBS as a side effect. Research is now investigating how the gut brain influences the immune system since 70 percent of our immune system is aimed at bacteria found in the gut.

The nerves of the gut brain allow the gastrointestinal (GI) tract to go beyond food digestion. With so many neurotransmitters involved in this location, it is no wonder that these signals affect other locations in the body - specifically the thinking brain and how we process life experiences. Serotonin and dopamine are two such examples tied to depression and mental well being. With approximately 90% and 50%, respectively, of both serotonin and dopamine produced in the gut - we can see why this psychological disorder is connected to the gut brain - as well as the primary treatments. Another great example is IBS, where mental stress often serves as a trigger for bowel symptoms.

Furthermore, the vagal nerves transmits information between the brain and the GI tract in both directions; specifically, regulating GI secretory, motor function, GI endocrine activity, and the sensations of satiety and sedation which are vagal responses. Though the vagal input and output is important for every day GI function, it does prove unnecessary. This is because the gut truly has a 'mind of its own' as it continues to function independently even if the vagal nerve input is severed or stopped. The complex interactions of the GI system, its neurotransmitters, and the rest of the body - including the brain - is quite complex and is still undergoing further studies to better understand these systems. The vagus nerve serves as the prime parasympathetic component contributing to the body's homeostasis.

As previously mentioned, this controls the "rest and digest" element of our autonomic nervous system allowing the body to better heal, relax, and absorb nutrients. The vagus nerve benefits impacts one's ability to decrease heart rate and respiratory rates, to regulate various glands within the body and improve digestive functioning. These aspects are performed subconsciously and continuously all day every day. Problems with hyperarousal, heart issues, digestive disorders, among other maladies, may occur when the vagus nerve and the parasympathetic system are not working properly. Furthermore, one's vagal tone correlates to how he or she may deal with and react to stressful stimuli.

Understanding all this is relative to how we react to stressful stimuli. As evidence has redundantly shown that stress has the potential to manifest into illness, by utilizing resilience practices, one can help prevent dysfunction within the body. On a cellular level, when our food is digested it is distributed through the body to serve as nourishment and an energy source. But when it isn't digested properly, it becomes a source of illness manifesting into constipation, heartburn, IBS, diarrhea, and other digestive issues.

This also correlates psychologically. When our experiences are not 'digested' in a proper way it becomes a dysfunction to our health and wellness. Whether these dysfunctions include self sabotage, overthinking, depleted self confidence, rash anger, manipulative behaviors, attachment to material items, or even depression- each imbalance can lead one to a self destructive path both within the body and beyond the body.

IBS and Stress

There is a clear psychological component to our digestion as we have just explored. If one experiences heartbreak or disappointment or horrible news, they may feel their stomach hurting, not have an appetite, or even have diarrhea. Similarly someone in love may experience the sensation of 'butterflies' within the stomach. Yogis have noted that when one has stomach pain by slow, deep breathing the pain can be redirected and flushed out of the body. Proper functioning on digestion relies so much on our nervous system, specifically our parasympathetic nervous system. This is where the term "rest and digest" comes from since relaxation facilitates better bowel function and stress attributes to pathologies such as IBS.

In the clinical setting, personal experience has shown that those affected by IBS often have an exacerbation of symptoms associated with stressful life events. Such potential emotional stressors could be a new medical diagnosis, losing a job, or a death in the family - among others. Stress can also present in other forms such as with food intolerances. In those intolerant of any type of food - often spicy foods, carbonation, alcohol as well as various fruits and vegetables - the physical stress of the food's inability to be properly digested can trigger IBS symptoms. Chemical and hormonal stressors, such as seen in menstruation, likely also correlate as well, noting that females are twice as likely to experience IBS.

Addie came to yoga to shed some pounds and work on stress management. At age 56 she had been divorced 4 years earlier and was still holding resentment for her failed marriage. The pent up feelings initiated stress making it difficult to move on and feel whole again. After a couple of sessions, she began asking me questions regarding her diet because she wrestled with constipation. Pairing her digestive issues with her source of stress, we began working on letting go of things in her personal life that she couldn't change. Using Mindfulness Based Stress Reduction practices and yoga for digestive health, Addie began releasing her resentment, guilt, and hurt from the divorce which alleviated the constipation. We began to shift her energy from dwelling on the emotional pain to attending the present and building the tools for her to orchestrate healing. Addie is still maintaining her home practice as she continues to nourish herself from the inside. She was able to shed some of the physical weight through muscle strengthening and stress reduction all while providing her a new mental framework of hope for the joy in her coming days.

Depression

Depression occurs when depleted norepinephrine cause flatness, apathy, or poor concentration. Decreased dopamine and serotonin levels lead to a lack of ability to experience pleasure, drive, and curiosity about life. Globally, more than 350 million people suffer from depression and depression is the leading illness in adults often occurring with other health maladies. The current medical treatment for depression is the use of antidepressants, but unfortunately possess many common side effects. Antidepressants more so numb the individual rather than addressing the source of pain or deficiency. The medication does not necessarily bring out feelings of joy, but has been shown to improve quality of life.

The third chakra correlates with our energy and when off balanced, whether there is too much energy or not enough, illnesses like depression or symptoms of complacency may occur. Yoga purposes the space to meet yourself where you are; showing up with your whole self. Your angry self if you are angry, your sad self if you are sad, your joyful self if you have joy, and even your empty self if you feel empty. It is a process of recognizing and accepting. From there, transformation can occur. One study suggests that three months of practicing yoga for ninety minutes a week improved depression participants by fifty percent. Other studies have shown the significance of savasana (relaxation pose at the end of yoga) for depression along with illustrating decreased self-reported symptoms of depression and anxiety, higher cortisol levels than the control group, and improved mood within young adults.

From a yogic perspective, depressed people often do not have enough energy because they are disconnected from their breath causing shallow breathing. Inhalation produces energy while exhales relax the body. A slumped over posture may also make it hard to access this energy because the chest is so closed off inhibiting breath capacity. Heart opening stretches create more space within the chest expanding lung capacity, deepening the breath, and improving posture. When we breathe deeply we enrich our mind and body with a fresh, cleansing capability to release the stale disturbances that may have been created by unhealthy environments or dysfunctional feelings. The ancient Yogis understood that through conscious breath regulation you can manage your feelings and moods by increasing the energy within your body or by slowing the breath and relaxing. To experience our direct ability to influence how we feel and to heal is not only empowering, but also an innate sustainable mechanism to living a quality life.

Another reported symptom in depression is the lack of connection one may feel with his or her surroundings. By cultivating a connection with what is inside opens the gateway to creating these connections on the outside. It is about connecting with the community within. Through meditation, self care, and patience we can re-channel our quality of thought towards ourselves and our environment creating a new thought platform regarding how we feel, what we enjoy, and who we are. We must remember, even in these deep releases of grief and suffering, to consciously acknowledge our gratitude for the enormous capacity to feel.

Self Healing Tools

Mind

Reflecting back on second chakra in terms of facing pain or challenges with a fresh perspective, empowers our ability to cope with life experiences and circumstances that may trigger depression. Through mindful practices such as yoga nidra and self awareness, one can paint acceptance within the heart to cultivate a natural way to self-sustainability in resilience and healing. This goes back to meeting yourself where you are. Know that it is okay if you do not have energy to go to a class. Start slowly. Motivation to the mat begins with the mind.

Light Visualization

Lying in a comfortable position, allow the eyes to close. Notice the natural breath traveling in and out of the body. Take a moment to follow that breath. Notice how the body softens, relaxing the legs, the hips, the belly, the chest, the arms, the face, the eyes. Feel the body become weightless as though you could float away. On your next inhale, begin to infuse the body with light. As this light begins to fill the low belly with detached awareness, witness how it illuminates up into the forehead- hold. Maybe imagine feeling warmth here in your forehead. As you exhale, slowly notice as the light absorbs deeper into the body. Inhale, feeling the light expand throughout the body- imagining the warm sensations into the toes to the fingertips. Exhale, softening into the light. Inhale as the light emulates throughout the entire body. Flow here with your natural breath and this visualization of light resounding within you. Imagining you are a weightless pillow of light.

Meditation (pg. 102)

Mindfulness (pg. 106)

Body

See Yoga Glossary for Third Chakra Yoga Poses

Lying down poses are the best to begin for healing depression so maybe begin lying down on your back. Draw your knees into your chest and rock side to side. Close your eyes and tune into the sensations you feel within the body. Not judging, but just witness how your body feels in this moment. Notice how the breath flows effortlessly out of the nose and into the nose. Soften the face, the jaw, the belly. Imagine the entire body being enveloped by complete calm. Now, take a deep breath in and infuse the body with light. Hold the breath and feel the light expanding throughout your chest and through your whole body. Gently exhale letting your hands open and relax. Inhale, infuse the body with light and exhale to receive light. Follow your breath and allow the body to relax. If any thoughts arise notice them as if they are leaves and sticks floating down a river stream.

Starting slow is imperative to healing, giving time time. Slow, gentle movements aligned with the breath revitalize the nervous system. Backbends energize the body and as BKS Iyengar once said "Keep your arms above your head, you cannot be depressed with your armpits open." Lifting the eyes and sun salutations have been shown to improve mood and energy.

Tapping

Tapping, also known as Emotional Freedom Technique (EFT), is based on the energy meridians used in traditional acupuncture to treat emotional and physical maladies by using the fingertips to input kinetic energy onto specific acupressure points. Tapping on these points can release pain, fears, and negative emotions that are stored within the body. When the meridians are stimulated, the amygdala receives the message of safety, thus causing it to calm down. The amygdala acts like a sensor within the limbic brain that goes off when it interprets a threat. The hippocampus validates the amygdala by confirming or denying if a true threat is present; however, in chronic stress, the hippocampus cannot shut off the amygdala causing a state of hyper arousal within the body as seen with PTSD. Tapping is a wonderful method to comfort and calm the amygdala enveloping safety and peace into the body and mind. It is a way to provide feedback from meridian cues shutting off the stress response and generates the parasympathetic nervous system to envelope the system. Tapping is a form of psychological acupressure and when thinking of your specific fear, trauma, or circumstance paired with voicing positive affirmations- healing is awakened within the mind and body.

Whether facing depression or anxiety, this technique is an effective way to break through blocks within the body and affirm empowerment and safety to have optimal mental and physical health. If facing an anxiety attack or stress, tapping is especially good for grounding and calming the body and mind back into balance.

An exercise I use, especially if a patient comes to me overwhelmed and anxious we begin tapping as soon as they start expressing their troubles moving from crown of the head, above the eyebrows, temple, cheek bone, above the lip, chin, chest, and sides of the body. Speaking to the pain you feel is a transformational way of healing yourself. So for instance, as my patient expresses their fears or situation, they follow along with me tapping the meridians. Once they are finished expressing themselves they repeat after me an affirmation such as, "Even though I have all this pain, I deeply and completely love and accept myself."

How to Tap

It doesn't matter how fast or slow you tap,
find a pace that feels right for you.

*For depression or lack of excitement,
motivation, and zest for life:*

Beginning with finding a comfortable position,
simply begin noticing initially how your body
feels. Do not judge it or acknowledge the source for
your discomfort but witness how you feel.

Begin by using both hands tapping with your fingertips onto
the crown of your head- take a deep breath in and sigh it out.
Move your fingertips tapping onto the forehead-
take a deep breath in and sigh it out.
Move your fingertips tapping onto your temples-
take a deep breath in and sigh it out.
Move your fingertips tapping onto your cheekbones-
take a deep breath in and sigh it out.
Move your dominant hand fingertips tapping right
above the lip- take a deep breath in and sigh it out.
Move both hands with fingertips tapping on your
chin- take a deep breath in and sigh it out.
Move your fingertips tapping down to your
chest- take a deep breath in and sigh it out.
Cross your arms and gently 'karate chop' or tap the
sides of your torso (and if you prefer to do one side that
is fine too)- take a deep breath in and sigh it out.

Practice this for two-five rounds and then once you are
finished, close your eyes. Begin to notice the sensations you feel
within your body. Notice if you can feel the rhythm pulsating
through your body. Take a deep breath in and sigh it out. Give
yourself permission to not know all the answers but to simply
feel what is in this moment now. You can now move into a
meditation practice if you like or simply relax where you are.

For anxiety, fear, pain, trauma, chronic stress,
or feelings of overwhelmed stress:

Beginning with a comfortable position, begin to notice
how you feel and where your distress is coming from.

Start with speaking about your negative feelings using
this moment to voice how you feel for ventilation.
As you voice your feelings or address your pain, begin
tapping on the outside of your hand where you would "karate
chop" something. It doesn't matter which hand you start
with, tap the outside of you hand- voicing how you feel.
Move to your wrists by tapping your wrists
together- voicing how you feel
Now bring both hands tapping with your fingertips
onto the crown of your head- voicing how you feel.
Move your fingertips tapping onto the
forehead- voicing how you feel.
Move your fingertips tapping onto your
temples voicing how you feel.
Move your fingertips tapping onto your
cheekbones- voicing how you feel.
Move your dominant hand fingertips tapping
right above the lip- voicing how you feel.
Move both hands with fingertips tapping
on your chin- voicing how you feel.
Move your fingertips tapping down to
your chest- voicing how you feel.
Cross your arms and gently 'karate chop' or tap
the sides of your torso (and if you prefer to do one
side that is fine too)- voicing how you feel.

Do this for as long as it takes to flush out what doesn't
serve you. Once you feel you have nothing else to
say regarding your feelings or discomfort. Now we
will begin releasing through affirmation.

Begin with the outside of your hand tapping-
"Even though I feel all this pain"
Now move to your wrists by tapping your wrists together-
"I deeply and completely love and accept myself"

Bring both hands tapping with your fingertips onto the
crown of your head- "Through my breath I can release it."
Move your fingertips tapping onto the forehead-
"Through my affirmations I can let it go."
Move your fingertips tapping onto your
temples- "I can release this pain I feel."
Move your fingertips tapping onto your cheekbones-
"My pain will not hold me captive."
Move your dominant hand fingertips tapping right
above the lip- "I am not a prisoner of my pain."
Move both hands with fingertips tapping on your
chin- "I am ready to release my pain."
Move your fingertips tapping down to your chest- "I
can breathe more easily and feel liberation."
Cross your arms and gently 'karate chop' or tap the
sides of your torso (and if you prefer to do one side that
is fine too)- "I am free, letting go of this pain."

You can practice the releasing process as many times as
you would like. If you do not feel better, try tapping in each
part longer. Once you are finished- rest your arms and close
your eyes. Feel the sensations within your body. This is you
nurturing you. This is you healing you. To heighten your
relaxation, follow the sensations you feel into meditation.
Or simply honor yourself, listening to the wisdom of your
body to guide you into the next step for self care.

Acupuncture and Acupressure

As a medical student and resident physician, I (KH) was only
taught traditional Western medicine. Many of my patients were
taking over a dozen separate medications - many of which were
unnecessary. Rather than provide an external solution in the
form of a pill or injection, I wanted to find an intrinsic method
of treatment to reduce both medical costs as well as dependency

on medications. That was when I learned about acupuncture and acupressure.

Admittedly, I was skeptical at first, but kept an open mind as I learned about these treatment modalities. Once my certification was complete, I began offering acupuncture and acupressure treatments to my patients. Many were just as skeptical as I, but decided to try anyways. The majority who tried these nontraditional treatments enjoyed a decrease in chronic pain, migraines, joint aches, a muscle stiffness - among other complaints. Though these treatment modalities are not for all patients, I have experienced dozens of success stories in my clinic where patients have been able to reduce or eliminate the use of opioids or other analgesics.

Breath

Square Breathing

Square breathing is a pranayama exercise that utilizes equal breath count in four parts. This practice is calming and meditative promoting balance within the body and rejuvenates the nervous system.

To begin take a deep breath in, sigh it out.

Slowly in half for 1, 2, 3, 4. Hold the breath in the forehead for 1, 2, 3, 4. Slowly exhale for 1, 2, 3, 4. Hold the breath in the belly for 1, 2, 3,4.

Continue this for at least one minute.

As you practice and increase your breath capacity, you may draw out the breath for five or six counts rather than four.

Breath of Fire

Breath of Fire, also known as Kapilabhati, forces full exhalation and a passive inhalation which helps stimulate the solar plexus, quickly oxygenates blood, strengthens the nervous system, and strengthens both lung capacity and respiratory functioning.

If you have high blood pressure, suffering from a severe respiratory infection, abdominal ulcers, diabetes, or are pregnant it is best to refrain from this breathing technique. It is also not recommended for those who suffer from cardiac problems or spinal disorders.

Begin sitting up straight allowing the shoulders to relax back. You want to equalize the length of your inhales and exhales, however, the exhale requires more tonic energy where the inhale is passive. This practice is done by pumping the navel out as you exhale, breathing rapidly. Using your fingers to snap setting the pace like a metronome helps with concentration in this pranayama exercise.

HEART CHAKRA

Love Thyself

"There is one word which may serve as a rule of practice for all one's life - reciprocity." - Confucius

The heart chakra is the fourth of the chakras located in the cardiac and pulmonary plexus. The hormones and glands located here are the heart peptides and thymus gland, which is partly responsible for the immune system. Anahata is the Sanskrit word meaning "unstruck" delineating the notion 'of that which you cannot attack'. This is the place of self-understanding where one chooses what serves them and what doesn't. Furthermore, empowering one to lay down boundaries through participating in lifestyle choices and habits that are healthy. When the third chakra is in balance it directs energy up into the heart stimulating the desire to serve and make positive choices. Activities and attitudes that support the heart chakra, which also improving one's immunity and wellness include: hope, forgiveness, humility, agape love, service, and self-care. As immunity physically exists in the body, when we keep ourselves well, there is also a metaphysical existence of immunity emulated within this chakra. When someone realizes unhealthy lifestyle choices or relationships present in their life and chooses to let those things that are unhealthy go; they are participating in immunity. We often times poison ourselves by our own choices, but when we practice this idea of letting go what doesn't serve us- it is then we can heal ourselves and maintain wellness.

When one accesses the heart chakra, he or she has overcome preoccupations of lower chakra tendencies with improved concentration, ethics and morals. This space of self-understanding is where one is aware of their goals, actions, and role in life actively participating in the greater good. Imbalances present in the heart chakra may look like codependency, arrogance, an inability to forgive, burnout, reactive anger, fear and greed. Other characteristics of the heart chakra are freedom, the color of smoky green, the element of air, self control, the sense of touch, serving others, giving guidance, compassion, nurturing, self confidence, passions that are tamed, holding healthy boundaries, and fearlessness.

Service is a prominent behavior expressed through this chakra as the hands and arms are an extension of this chakra. But for service to maintain healthy, giving must come from a place of containment. Not giving too much of oneself which could lead to burnout or co-dependency, but the ability to say no. Martin Luther King Jr. is a great example of the heart chakra because he saw something present in his community that was hurting and not serving for the better good and he stood up saying, "No, I will not tolerate this" and served to make a change. The shadow of the heart is reactive anger, however, when we act out of controlled anger this becomes a catalyst to something great. Boundaries are very healthy and are necessary for one to maintain the 'knowing what is me and what isn't me'. Giving too much or not giving at all can lead to several imbalances in our lives and relationship.

Stress and the Heart

In the discussion of the second chakra and trauma, we touched base with stress and its effects within the body. As noted, our cuddle hormone, oxytocin, is released during our stress response. Kelly McGonigal noted in her Ted Talk 'How to make Stress your Friend' that by our means of caring we create resiliency and that we must address how stress gives us access to our hearts. The American Heart Association has done a wonderful job with raising awareness about heart disease and the effects of stress and lifestyle choice. By what we feed ourselves, environment, work conditions, and stress can contribute deeply to our heart health. It is imperative to address the effects of stress on heart health and by contouring our attitude towards stress can build the resilience necessary to abolish the negative effects stress can have on our heart.

"Above all else, guard your heart, for everything you do flows from it." Proverbs 4:23

Our stress response is inherently designed to manage stress. The yoga practice has an incredible way to shape our thought forms of stress as something temporary or that the challenges we face is essentially our curriculum to evolve. We must understand that there is something beautiful yielded from the hard times. Whether it is a refined heart or transforming that pain into wisdom- we learn something new about ourselves that can enhance our understanding of the bigger picture. Grief and suffering do not just change an individual, but it becomes a revelation of one's deepest self. And as each trial surfaces, we strengthen our resilience. In my yoga classes, sometimes as I have my students practice balancing poses, I remind them to embrace the wiggle room. The wiggle room-where we may fall, wobble, or hop around- is the curriculum. It is through our imbalance that we may learn how to source balance. The wiggle room teaches what serves and what doesn't. And when we fall, we are faced with the choice to either give up or try again. We face that choice everyday. Each time we try again we create another layer of resiliency. Furthermore, it teaches us to not be afraid of falling. No successful business didn't have a trial and error time or make mistakes. The most successful individuals have had some sort of refining moment in their life or a traumatic experience that transformed them into a better, wiser version of themselves. In life we must let go of striving for perfection, but strive for connection. It is through this practice that we create resilience.

So when we become overwhelmed or stressed out, oxytocin is released. This hormone fine tunes our social instincts and instills the desire to connect with others. This is what motivates one to vent or seek support during difficult times. As McGonigal states that our biological responses tell us that "We do not have to face stress alone." Self care practices, group therapy, friendship, and/ or other resources that create the opportunity for us to connect deeper with ourselves and others have shown to improve heart health and higher resilience to stress. There have also been some great studies out there about the positive impact on our health from serving others such as a longer lifespan, greater self worth and meaning, lower blood pressure, better pain management, and overall happiness.

Within the Yoga Sutras, Patanjali discusses the Four Keys to Peace in Sutra 33. He writes, "By cultivating attitudes of friendliness toward the happy, compassion for the unhappy, delight in the virtuous, and disregard toward the wicked, the mind-stuff retains its undisturbed calmness." Often times we can lose our peace over the attitudes and behaviors of the individuals in our lives- especially when it comes to individuals we love. But by practicing these attitudes towards circumstances where an individual may be representing one of these "locks," you will have the "key" to respond maintaining serenity within the mind, furthermore, protecting the heart from stress and burnout.

The first lock is the happy person and the key to this individual is friendliness. As Nelson Mandela once said, "Resentment is like drinking poison and then hoping it will kill your enemies." We must be mindful to never have an attitude of resentment or jealousy towards a happy person, rather, meet that happy person with friendliness. The second lock is the unhappy person and the key to this individual is compassion. We have all been unhappy at times in our lives. When someone is upset, comfort them. As mentioned earlier, caring creates resilience. Others can take strength from our stories or even just our presence can be really healing for an unhappy person. But at the same time, respecting both your boundaries and their boundaries. Always offer compassion. Never take pleasure in someone's suffering. As the saying goes, "The only time you should look down on someone, is when you are helping them up."

The next lock Patanjali discusses is virtuous people. The key to virtuous people is delight. As quoted, "Don't envy him; don't try to pull him down. Appreciate the virtuous qualities in him and try to cultivate them into your own life." Noble people inspire our own horizons to expand so we may also offer ourselves to serve or live in virtue, then in return ignite these qualities into others. Through this process we can clothe ourselves in these virtues to become a better, more refined version of ourselves equipped with the wisdom and resilience to overcome suffering and let go of the things no longer serving in our lives.

The last lock is the wicked person. As none of us are perfect, there are times where we encounter or may be that wicked person. Whether the individual is someone who challenges your values, hurts others, or hurts themselves- the key to this behavior is disregard. This is the hardest, especially when it is someone we love or somebody we may feel is 'out to get us'. I remember growing up my mother always told me when somebody was picking on me, to ignore them and they will become bored and move on to someone else. Furthermore, Patanjali warns that advising a wicked person will result in the loss of peace. We can only control our own actions and our own reactions. Life has an interesting way of teaching people and Patanjali expresses that he or she will have to learn by experience. These 'keys' hold the power to maintain peace of mind and a serene heart.

It is important to maintain awareness that our attitudes, emotions, and thoughts can have an effect on our health. It is a balance between the will and strength to show up attending whatever circumstance may arise and to surrender into the experience. If each moment is our current assignment, let us use it to grow, to heal, and to be refined. On the yoga mat for instance, when we are challenged with a strengthening pose that may be uncomfortable or difficult, practicing softening in the body, relaxing the face, and breathing slow in and out the nose rewires the brain to better soften and relax when faced with discomfort or stress off the mat. We don't just build physical stamina but improve our experiences when facing stress.

Fatigue/Burn Out

Fatigue and burnout are often triggered by dysfunctional movement patterns that wreak havoc on the body, render shortness of breath, induce stress- all usually stemmed from over doing it. We are a culture that is constantly plugged in and on the go. Eventually, at some point, when there is no self-care or maintenance implemented into the week, we "burn out." This causes increased exhaustion, sensitivity to stress, weight gain, migraines, anxiety, and other health ailments. Furthermore, our productivity, attention to detail and overall quality of life plummets. I love the saying "When you start to trim the leaves, it blooms" because abundance will flow when we simplify things and clarify what is important. This relates to letting go of what doesn't serve you- even if that means leaving a job, stepping away from a group of friends or even getting out of a toxic relationship. Giving yourself to everything and showing up for everyone will make you sick. Create space for yourself to recharge or you will compromise the quality of how you show up for life.

Implementing small life style changes and practices throughout your day can make a huge difference. Whether creating more time for yourself in the mornings, cutting out extraneous activities that may be taking away time from things that are more important, or by simply saying no; we must set boundaries in order to return and maintain a necessary balance. Many of my clients will justify their burnout by claiming how there 'just isn't enough time'. So many people give all their power up to a clock or use it to justify complacency and fear, when in reality, life truly only exists in the present moment. Invite yourself to break down the limitations set up in your mind and begin to listen to what you truly need in the present moment. Balance in the heart chakra consists of being open to both giving and receiving. If we are just giving and giving and giving we will eventually burn out and become sick. To make time for yourself is an opportunity to practice healthy, self love and cultivate the energy to provide more value when we show up for others.

Fatigue and burnout may also be the consequence from the illusion of competition or that 'there isn't enough for me'. A balanced heart chakra understands abundance. A balanced heart chakra sees that there is always enough and that competition is simply the shadow of the heart. When we are driven by competition, our achievements no longer hold authenticity to universal love and abundance. It causes division and separates us from achieving our uniquely, individualized purpose. Your purpose is yours. When one door closes another opens if you choose to knock. If you didn't get the job you wanted or the 'thing' you hoped for, knock and ask for what you want. Be clear, but be balanced. There is enough for everyone. You are already enough.

Jenna, 32, was the director of a music program for one of the local universities and spent much time each day of the week working late into the evenings. When she would get off work, she would prepare her music programs and classes for the following day. When Jenna came to yoga, she was very critical of herself. Often she would cry as soon as she arrived as a result of being so exhausted and overwhelmed. Many times she would cancel due her fear of not having enough time to fit her self care in. Our classes were very restorative, meditative flow, heart opening, and meditation based. In the beginning she was very resistant to doing anything outside of our sessions because she feared she wouldn't have time, but would rave about how wonderful she felt after the session and into the next day. Jenna would go above and beyond for her students at the university she worked for along with the volunteer work she did, but would leave feeling depleted and anxious. Her chaotic lifestyle was causing her to gain weight and feel depressed. In our sessions we began addressing self care and self love. By implementing daily affirmations, Jenna began to feel grounded and nurtured before she started her day. After six weeks, Jenna began cutting back in her job and requesting the university to hire someone to help her out with the music program. Jenna now feels more organized, practices yoga on her own, and has begun creating daily affirmations for herself to generate self love. When Jenna began working with me she spoke so negatively about herself and now exemplifies confidence in her demeanor, has lost some weight, and is assertive about setting boundaries for herself.

When we do not take the measures necessary to care for ourselves, our drive shifts into overwhelm, avoidance, and/or resentment which could all lead to illness. Increased emotional stress, anger, and burnout have been linked to increased cardiovascular disease morbidity and mortality. In addition, there are associations with metabolic syndrome, hypothalamic-pituitary-adrenal axis dysregulation, sleep disturbances, inflammation, impaired blood coagulation and fibrinolysis, and poor health behaviors.

Furthermore, burnout decreases the effectiveness of one's immune system and ability to fight off infections. One example is through differences in vaccination responses from normal individuals and those experiencing burnout. Specifically, individuals with more stress and anxiety showed a delay in the immune response to the vaccine (or showed no response). In everyday life, this correlates to adults experiencing higher rates of clinical illness (Burns & Goodwin, 1990). Additionally, this is worrisome as those with burnout are at higher risk of suffering from more severe impairment in the face of common viruses and bacteria - causing more morbidity/mortality than experienced by the general populace. It costs an individual more to neglect their self care and health, than it would to simply take three minutes of meditation or just say no.

High Blood Pressure and Yoga

Often, the stress response to an overwhelming situations creates a desire to self loathe or medicate in order to soothe the trigger. By feeding into this desire, it can lead to negative coping mechanisms that are counterintuitive to healing and restoring energy. Excessive fat, alcohol, or television use may feel good in the moment, however, they actually have no positive effect on the long term issues and worsen one's health with prolonged use. Let us take hypertension as an example. Approximately one in three people have high blood pressure - leading to almost 40 million hospital and clinic visits annual for this condition. Though most do not experience symptoms from hypertension, the evidence shows that this "silent killer" should be controlled via appropriate lifestyle choices and medications if warranted. If left untreated over prolonged periods, hypertension will decrease one's quality of life and is associated with numerous other pathologies like stroke, heart attacks, and kidney disease.

The higher the pressure within the heart, the greater the strain on optimal functionality. Symptoms like lightheadedness or headaches may be the body's red flag warning of too much pressure within the heart- the lower the pressure, the better because it is easier on the heart and blood vessels. Optimal blood pressure is under 120/80, however, blood pressure fluctuates throughout each day. If an individual is anxious, blood pressure may rise. In clinical settings, often times whether it be due to patient anxiety over being seen by the doctor or a patient in physical pain, the readings for blood pressure may be inaccurate due to this known as "white-coat hypertension." The best time to get an accurate reading on your blood pressure is by taking the measurements yourself in your home.

Often times, readings for high blood pressure may not have a known cause. This is known as "essential hypertension" which is unconnected from blood pressure that is elevated due to serious health problems. Identifying the underlying cause for essential hypertension can often be sourced from prescription drugs, stress, steroids, and nasal decongestants. If a patient's blood pressure is high, most medical experts recommend giving non-drug interventions before actually prescribing medication, unless a reading that is high shows evidence of damage to the heart and/ or kidneys.

It is well known that diet, exercise, and stress management plays a vital role in maintaining a healthy BP. Sustained stress levels can lead to hypertension, therefore, beginning with ways to eliminate stress may help reduce the risk and improve blood pressure. Furthermore, when someone is under a lot of stress, they are more likely to smoke cigarettes, develop dysfunctional eating habits, develop sleep disorders, and drink alcohol which can contribute to high blood pressure. Yoga and mindfulness have been shown to reverse these tendencies and instill healthy coping mechanisms in the face of stress and can lessen a person's level of pain - which directly affects blood pressure. Additionally, it seems that mindfulness and yoga can generate a peace of mind that motivates an individual to take better care of themselves cultivating a deeper connection within the mind and body relationship.

Although many studies show yoga and mindfulness having a modest, but consistent decrease in blood pressure, these modest changes may have a significant effect on reducing the chances of stroke and heart disease. More controlled research and evidence will need to be conducted to show further evidence for yoga being a treatment method for hypertension, however, it is suggested that yoga and mindfulness are effective when incorporated for prevention of hypertension and heart disease.

Aadil Palkhivala, an Ayurvedic physician and yoga therapist, has conducted much work and research around the effectiveness of holistic intervention and hypertension. He teaches that hypertension is divided into two categories; the first being where the nervous system is exhausted and therefore jittery. The second categories exemplifies those who are metaphorically stuck which causes the nervous system to pent up energy. Palkhivala believes when it comes to yoga, the two types should be addressed differently to create proper balance within the body. A patient under the jittery HBP category are often overworked and consistently on the go. More restorative and mindfulness with calming breathing techniques embedded into the yoga practice allows the nervous system to restore itself and recuperate optimum energy. On the contrary, a patient who can be categorized under pent up HBP have less motion in their lives and experiences feelings of frustration and complacency. Utilizing a vigorous, fluid yoga practice allows the pent up pressure to disperse throughout the body, while also honing into stretching the muscles out.

It is no surprise the body is most healthy in homeostasis, hence we should always strive for balance. Understanding how our relationships, work environment, and feelings can affect our health is crucial to address in order to obtain wellness. Too much of anything is never good, so moderating our stagnancy and our pace will allow us to generate a lifestyle that supports what we truly need in order to thrive.

Self Healing Tools

Mind

Forgiveness

There have been many variations of the quote anger, resentment, or not forgiving is like drinking poison yourself and waiting for the other person to die. This aphorism expresses the reality of holding onto anger and hurt, rather than letting go. The inability to forgive inhibits you from living. Not forgiving will make you sick. I (MA) began working with Jackie after her husband had returned from his second tour to Afghanistan. All of Jackie's life she made all effort to control each agent within her life. In our initial consultation together, she made it clear what kind of sequence she wanted and the exact number of pounds she was going to lose. Her stubborn attitude of 'my way or the highway' was her way of protecting herself and had become a survival tactic to alleviate disappointment. As Jackie was very stern and appeared confident in her demeanor, after a few weeks she began to open up to the circumstances that she couldn't control enraged and acting from the victim archetype. Through these discussions she exemplified a lot of anger and hatred towards people and things that didn't go her way. Her husband "wasn't the same" anymore so she hated the Army. She hated her son's fiancee with no substance of reason. She blamed her mother for her own challenges. Blaming and hating her mother, her son's fiance, and the Army was only hurting Jackie. Jackie had a very shallow breath and her chest muscles were so tight that her upper back and shoulders were rounded. We began using loving kindness meditations and practicing radical forgiveness.

During our yoga sequences, we worked on discharging Jackie's pent up anger and energy to ease the nervous system and soften into difficult poses along with practicing heart openers and breathing exercises to deepen and slow her breath. After three months of working together, Jackie was much softer in her demeanor and began attending military spouse support meetings with others who were dealing with similar circumstances as she was. She became open to spending time with her son's fiance and continued practicing loving kindness towards those that she was hurt by and accepting the things that did not measure up to her expectations.

Life is unpredictable and we must accept there are going to be things that we have no control over. Practicing both forgiveness of others and forgiveness towards ourselves opens a new possibility to sustainable peace and happiness. Expectation is the thief of love. Be present and breathe with the moment, whether it is uncomfortable or natural we must learn to adapt and retain the experience as a lesson. Never a mistake.

Body

See Yoga Glossary for Fourth Chakra Poses

Body and Breathing

When you own your breath nobody can steal your peace. -Unknown Author

The heart chakra's element is air found in both the heartbeat itself and through respiration. The breath has an overwhelming influence on the nature of the body. Each inhalation and exhalation interconnects with the nervous system and is the flame that either ignites a sympathetic response or the anchor that orchestrates a parasympathetic response. Our lungs help regulate the body's pH and maintain a proper blood acidity compatible for living. Breathing can affect lymph circulation which pumps from the thymus gland, heart rate variability, blood pressure, and cognitive functioning. Depending on the quality of breath, your breath can cultivate either a negative or positive effect within the body. Meditative flow yoga, for example, where the movement is initiated by the breath while the mind is focused on the breath generates a movement relationship that helps not only stretch the muscles that may be responsible for bad posture but also it connects one deeper to the breath.

Furthermore, opening the heart (stretching the chest muscles, strengthening upper back muscles) creates more space for the breath improving lung capacity. Rounded shoulders or a slump posture cuts off deep breathing and restricts the pulmonary volume. Take a moment, notice your seated posture. Maybe your shoulders are rounded forward and the chest is tight, closing over the heart space. It can lead to an irritable, icky feeling that may collect in the chest. Some describe it as heaviness in the chest or a feeling of combustion - like frustration. The way we carry ourselves can have a large impact on our energetic demeanor. An erect, strong posture transmits happiness and confidence whereas slouching postures portray the opposite. Furthermore, with this awareness we can employ specific movements to rejuvenate the body and return to balance.

Below is a great practice to 'break open the chest' and to create more space for breath expelling that icky feeling to elicit clarity and peace.

Begin sitting in Indian style. Take your hands onto your knees. (right hand on right knee, left hand on left knee). Take a deep breath in through the nose, and as you exhale, draw the left shoulder down and across the the body diagonally as if you are taking the left shoulder to touch the right knee. Inhale, come back up to center. Exhale, right shoulder dips down towards the left knee. Inhale come back up to center. Exhale left shoulder towards right knee. Inhales lift you as the exhales draw the shoulder across the body towards the opposite knee. Continue this at your pace. As you practice this meditative flow- if you begin to crave free movement, you can begin to move freely pivoting from the pelvis 'drawing circles with your heart' or any free movement that feels good opening the chest. Listen to the wisdom of your body, your body already knows what it needs.

We must acknowledge the important contribution respiration plays in the way we feel and how our lack of mobility can prompt dysfunction. When we have dysfunctional breathing, less oxygen enters the body and carbon dioxide escapes slower - derailing proper functioning and can lead to both emotional and physical ailments. As someone once stated, "Breathe. That is the wisest one word sentence." Whether one is breathing in a restorative pose, through the yoga practice, or throughout the day; quality breathing softens our physiology, keeping the heart healthy with a clear mind. Over time, the mindful, slow nostril breathing becomes second nature.

Breath and Prana

Prana and breath are interrelated in terms of sourcing our energy. Where one holds the breath within the body expounds energetic blocks or liberation and it is through the quality of our breath that maintains wellness, not necessarily the volume. Prana is the bridge between mind and body. Prana is energy. The term "yogi" essentially translates as the one whose energy is contained within the spine. Prana takes no shape but exists purely as energetic movement. We don't physically see breath, but we can feel it as a result of its transportation in and out of the body and the way it moves through us. This movement supports and sustains all the ways we function and can be categorized as the five prana vayus. Our natural breath communicates by its movement within us, whether it is only upper body or deep in the low belly. Quality breath flows from the top of the head down into the pelvic floor and back up again. Below we will briefly explore each category and its characteristics in relationship to our own healing and moving through energetic blocks that hold us from progressing towards optimal wellness. Prana vayus exemplify the currents of breath expression throughout the body.

Apana (Grounding Breath)

The movement of apana exists as a down and out force. We experience this as the pressure that creates menstruation, waste elimination, and birth. Energetically, apana plays a role in our ability to let go, forgive, or surrender. Abraham Hicks talks about how nothing you want is upstream. His analogy delineates that when we push against the organic current or river of our life we create suffering and challenge, but when we relax and trust the flow of providence we tend to discover that what we desired is downstream. Pushing against the current of life, such as fighting the things we cannot control, perpetuates suffering. This can create blocks in allowing life to unfold naturally. We can release the suffering by softening into surrender, letting go of the things that do not serve us, and grounding in this present moment. These simple attitudes can change our entire reality in relation to the problems that feel debilitating, especially those we have no control over.

This energy exists between the navel and pelvic floor. Apana is illustrated when our natural breath moves within our lower abdomen alone. Other than energetic adjustments in attitude, we can balance this through forward folding, hip opening, fluid movements, and inversions in the yoga practice. Meditation itself is the practice of surrender and can support our ability in shifting and releasing the block both physically and energetically. A balanced apana vayu is grounded and open.

Samana Vayu (Centering Breath)

The movement of samana exists as a contracting, in and down force located in the solar plexus. We experience this force through assimilation and digestion. Samana holds the third chakra characteristics of alchemy both physically and energetically. For example, when the body converts food into energy, when we digest our life experiences into wisdom, or convert information into knowledge. This process creates intelligence and clear perception. However, when our pain or experiences are not digested properly it weakens samana.

Samana can become imbalanced when we continue to take and carry experiences or energy that no longer hold value. Behaviors such as when one continues to make the same mistakes over and over again can create an energy clog within our lives. There is power to discrimination when we can take what has value and release what does not. Our gut feelings communicate a deeper level of knowing what serves us. When one neglects the body's communication, the breath can remain stuck in the abdomen creating feelings of being cemented and heavy. Balancing practices such as spinal twists, abdominal massage, and pranayama exercises can help move the prana throughout the body to revitalize one's energy. When samana is open one can experience more clarity and resilience within the mind and body.

Prana Vayu (Energizing Breath)

The movement of prana exists as an in and up, forwarding moving force. Prana is located within the mid chest and governs the inhalation. If prana is weak, we feel depleted and fatigued. Because prana relates to the inhale and builds with inhale retention, we can strengthen this space through receiving and recharging mentally and physically by self care and revitalizing our inner strength. The easiest way to identify if there is an imbalance within the prana vayu is through recognizing if one is burnt out; however, through adopting fourth chakra balancing one can source vitality to cure exhaustion. Sun salutations or energizing poses in the yoga practice can unfetter the block releasing the breath back up the body. By focusing on things that restore inner strength, the body can create the energy needed to thrive.

Udana Vayu (Ascending Breath)

The movement of udana exists as an up and out force correlated with exhalation. Udana corresponds with expression and inspiration all driven by our psychological evolution. Growth, will, determination, and inspiration fuels balance within the udana vayu. Imbalance is exemplified when one lacks expression or feels apathetic. Physiologically, the means of which we communicate occur through the udana force as air rises and passes through the larynx to produce speech or song. Cell growth is propelled by udana along with the movement of standing up or holding the head up literally and metaphorically. Those suffering with depression often have a block in the udana vayu and tend to hold their breath at the top of their chest.

Subtle considerations can strengthen the udana vayu by gazing up, lengthening the spine, and reaching towards the sky. In the meditation practice, visualizing expansive light and feeling the breath expand within the throat followed by a strong exhale out the nose is both soothing and allows the breath to move out rather than staying stuck within the throat. Flushing out the stagnant energy supports strong exhalations and balance within the udana vayu to maintain inspiration and expansion.

Vyana Vayu (Distributive Breath)

The movement of vyana is responsible for energy distribution throughout the body and exists as an outward, circular force integrating the core of the body with the extremities. Vyana pervades the whole body governing circulation, cardiac health, and the nervous system generating blood flow and pulsation. One's ability to emotionally process life experiences is also influenced and shows up as the way we circulate and move fluidly throughout various areas of our lives. Connecting all the vayus, vyana moves prana throughout the body keeping the circular channels clear and functioning.

Imbalance can translate through emotional behaviors and physical symptoms such as isolation, withdrawal, poor circulation, blocked arteries, and peripheral neuropathy. Movement and flow is key for keeping the vyana vayu functioning properly. Utilizing the yoga practice and poses that claim space operating with expanding movement into the extremities support circulation and energetic flow. By maintaining coordination and physical integrity, vyana can travel freely throughout the body preserving wellness, emotional freedom, and creativity.

By understanding how our breath can express symptoms of imbalance within the body, one can take subtle action to restore wellbeing. Movement is wellness and is imperative so the body may continue to move with optimal quality of breath. Our respiration is so innate to our existence that without it we do not survive. Although the breathing proves natural, it is easily neglected and with age it tends to founder. By adopting mindfulness and awareness of one's respirations, one can prevent malady simply by addressing subtle symptoms. The better we know our bodies, the better we can preserve wellness and heal ourselves.

THROAT CHAKRA

Bridging Mind and Body

"There is one whose rash words are like sword thrusts, but the tongue of the wise brings healing." Proverbs 12:18

The throat chakra is the fifth of the chakras located in the pharyngeal plexus, also known as the carotid plexus (cervical spine corresponding with the neck). The glands located here are the thyroid and parathyroid responsible for metabolism and calcium in the body. The vagus, glossopharyngeal, and sympathetic nerves are found in this region. And it is here where space and sound meet. An interesting way to think of the healing experience here is when sound and space meet it creates vibration stimulating a powerful parasympathetic response. This is why singing can be very soothing in the body and for the mind. Vishuddha is the Sanskrit word for "pure" represented by an expansive light blue. As we self-actualize, we remove impurities allowing confusion and constraints to dissolve. Space or ether represents the element for this chakra illuminating the expansiveness when one expresses or uses words to clarify an expression. The throat chakra is also where we manifest expression that is beyond words but through artistic and creative outlets.

Behavioral characteristics here are represented through communication, vibrancy, stillness, joy, peacefulness, and patience. There is a craving to seek knowledge and cultural conditioning while the predominant sense is hearing. Knowledge yields power, but can be used in creating doubt. However, through meditation, prayer, and experience one can alleviate doubt and the person becomes self-actualized. Imbalances here may appear as manipulation, suppressed thoughts, opinions, humiliation, lacking conviction behind your words, and emotional congestion. Expression is a way to purify our minds whether it is making sense of something or sharing a contributing thought or idea. This chakra accesses both creating and learning making it the catalyst to manifesting one's goals, dreams, and noble purpose. Furthermore, this chakra is associated with truth and living aligned with what you believe.

The throat chakra is the bridge between experience and expression - literally serving as the gateway between the body and the head. Maintaining balance means being affirmed in your right to speak or express thus moving it into action, impact, and connection. Our voice has influence when we believe what we have to say has meaning, but excessive talking dilutes the impact our voice can have. The throat chakra connects the heart and mind; therefore, the more clearly we understand what we need or what we feel- the better we utilize our voice as a catalyst for connection. Overly-thinking, self-criticism, and lying diminish our ability to be vulnerable and honest. The words and expressions we use cater to the great influence of how our life unfolds.

We become the artist of our lives through creation by the forms of which we express ourselves. As this is the location of our vocal chords - the method in which we speak with others- we can better understand why the throat chakra is attributed to any issues stemming from communication. The energy of our speech empowers us to share our desires and intentions to those around us. The power of one's voice should not be underestimated.

Power of Voice

Our voice is the conduit of our message. Voice is the vehicle that projects who we think we are, what we stand for, and how we can present our perceptions and truths to others. However, a man's tongue can can become the largest stumbling block. Jesus talked in the book of Matthew about how it is not what goes into the mouth that defiles the body, but what comes out. A balanced fifth chakra presents wisdom in words and uses this power for truth and good. As stress is the leading cause of many health problems today, when one has no control over their words it can lead to chaos in their life, thus manifesting into more stress, imbalance, and/or illness.

Integrative medicine breaks down the ailments to discover the source and invites one to reflect on the lifestyle choices that are impacting his or her health. So noticing tendencies that may cause imbalances such as being overly talkative and not listening to others, interrupting others when they are speaking, being overly aggressive in your opinions, or speaking false witness and lies. Most of these imbalances are due to reactivity in our emotion or beliefs. Meditation helps one create space between belief and doubt or emotion and reactivity helping transform judgement into compassion. Once we discipline our tendencies we are able to speak with power. Accessing this power begins with expressing ourselves effectively and keeping our conduct congruent to our words. By taking our power seriously, one can produce the tools, opportunities, and relationships to live the life he or she loves.

Melanie (47), growing up in an alcoholic home, at an early age developed a habit of suppression and lying. As a little girl, she would outwardly deny what was really going on at home and when talking to others, she would describe her home life very different from what it actually was. Overtime she found herself lying often about 'little things' and felt frustrated with herself. These frustrations led her to dysfunctional habits and would often surface in her relationships. When I began working with Melanie, she came to yoga to help better cope with stress. Five years previously she had a lobectomy (removal of half her thyroid) which took her many months to overcome fatigue and find some balance in her body. As we began working together, each session began with her explaining to me that everything is fine and she is happy- but once we began practicing, she would mention how her lower back has been bothering her or she feels frustrated with someone from work or that she was wounded by someone in her family. I noticed that Melanie had a hard time being clear on what she needed and felt she could not accurately create an intention for her practice. I began to give her homework to write daily affirmations and intentions along with different variations of bridge pose for her low back and thyroid. At first she was very hesitant with the affirmation writing practice but after a couple of weeks she began to really listen to what she needed and aligned her affirmations and intentions accordingly building her confidence in asking for what she needs. After five months of gentle, hatha flow yoga, five minute meditations, and working on affirmations; Melanie has been able to begin really transforming the way she speaks and the way she listens. She claims that her yoga practice has helped her feel more connected to herself and improved her feelings of feeling adequate.

Once we clearly understand what we need and what we stand for, abundance begins to flow due to our harmonic relationship with our bodies and life circumstances. This goes back to maintaining our boundaries, but also giving room to conserve the equilibrium of being heard and our ability to hear. The only witness to belief is action. Action must be manifested in order for balance to sustain and truth to transpire.

Sleep Apnea

Obstructive Sleep Apnea (OSA) is a medical condition where the upper airway relaxes during sleep and causes repetitive pauses in breathing and often an associated drop in oxygen levels in the blood. If severe enough, the individual will suffer from poor sleep, daytime fatigue, hypertension, and mood changes - among many other potential side effects. This is also associated with being overweight as one's neck girth tends to correlate with neck circumference. Along with weight or being stress induced, this condition may present in anyone, but is most common in those with large tonsils, smaller airways, and large necks. A common example is seen in the following case.

Tom (70), is a Vietnam veteran who came to me to address his weight and flexibility. He suffered from PTSD, insomnia, and sleep apnea. These conditions affected his nervous system where he would break out with rashes on his body and had a history of dealing with shingles. His weight was located in his stomach and it was clear this was caused by an over active nervous system. We began practicing yoga nidra twice a week paired with mediation and a gentle yoga practice once a week ending in relaxation and breathing exercises. Tom listened to a yoga nidra recording every night that helped him focus on his breathing and relaxation techniques guiding him to sleep. After 4 weeks, Tom's rashes began to clear up and he was beginning to have a few nights a week where he would sleep through the night without waking up. The yoga practice began to help strengthen and open Tom's body where he was feeling more energized and safe in his environment claiming he was "finally getting some peace of mind" and "looking forward to the next day." Tom also attended a local church and I asked him if he participated in the singing. He looked at me like I was crazy for asking this and replied laughing "what do you think?" I shared with him that singing actually may help strengthen the muscles in his throat and it could help with his sleep apnea. He shrugged it off and we continued our session. About a month later he told me he started to sing at church and even gave it a try while he was driving in his truck. He believed that it was actually helping because he hadn't awoken from not being able to breathe for almost a week. Tom has began meditating every morning, doing some stretches each day, and is feeling much more rested than he has in years.

Thyroid and Throat Chakra

The thyroid plays a vital role in our ability to feel and maintain health. It is quite common to have patients with dysfunctional thyroid glands - usually under-producing rather than over-producing thyroid hormones. This is a perfect example of how a single location can negatively affect the whole body when not functioning properly. Too little thyroid potentially leads to weakness, fatigue, weight gain, depression, cold intolerance, and dry skin - among many other symptoms. If overactive, the thyroid can cause sweating, fast heart rate, restlessness, and weight loss. In conjunction, the parathyroid consists of several small glands adjacent to the thyroid. Though its functions are different, the parathyroid can also over- or under-produce. A hyperactive parathyroid gland may cause kidney stones, altered mental status, increased urine output, dehydration, and increased risk of fractures. A hypoactive parathyroid may lead to muscle cramps, tingling sensations, irritability, and depression.

Both the thyroid and parathyroid often correlate directly with mood. Most people notice both physical as well as psychological consequences when one or both are functioning outside of the normal limits. Because of this known effect on the individual's mood, we can understand the biological relation of this chakra and our ability to express ourselves in relationship with our environment. Furthermore, a hypothyroid state can cause weight gain, hair loss, and skin changes - resulting in subsequent self image problems.

The thyroid plays a pivotal role throughout the body starting early in our lives, which contributes to multiple aspects of growth in the fetus. A hypothyroid state during this stage produces cretinism - characterized by severely stunted mental and physical development. Later in life, hypothyroidism still negatively affects multiple locations within body, though not as severely as in childhood, including mood, bowel movements, libido, depression, skin, and hair. When working correctly, the thyroid helps optimize psychological wellbeing, physical health, and healing in addition to ensuring that the throat chakra functions properly.

Beyond medical issues, this location can cause havoc on one's relationships - both at work and at home. I (KH) often hear concerns about relationship issues in couples that have otherwise had decades of wonderful years together. One of the labs I tend to check in this situation is thyroid function. Often times, hormone levels will be outside of regular limits to the point the patient requires medical intervention. Once thyroid function returns to normal, negative symptoms diminish and communication as well as the overall relationship may improve.

An imbalance in the throat chakra may be manifested through 'holding' or 'swallowing down.' Such examples may include holding onto an emotion and/or tendency or perhaps not cultivating an experience and/or disturbance into expression. Holding often times can result in weight gain because it may energetically disrupt our ability to control metabolism and secrete hormones properly. The ability to express feelings and truth simulates how we can release energy stored in the body that may be creating imbalances. It is important for those suffering with hypothyroidism practice speaking their truth. On contrary those with hyperthyroidism should practice listening more as imbalance may be sourced partially due to talking too much or talking over others.

As the thyroid impacts mood, attitude can play a large role in one's perceived happiness. Not only does a positive outlook improve day-to-day experiences, it also affects one's health in the long term. Positive psychology is a recent field founded on the belief that people want to live meaningful lives by cultivating the best versions of themselves. Happiness is enabled through avenues such as hope, creativity, wisdom, mindfulness, courage, spirituality, and perseverance which support an individual in overcoming negative impulses. By utilizing these avenues for expression and connection, individuals source the expression of the meaning they have created and process their life experiences. Optimism and hope on a cellular level can reconstruct thought platforms and develop optimal self-regulation patterns. In turn, positive psychology teaches that uplifting emotions broaden an individual's thought action receptors creating sustainable lifestyle choices.

Hypothyroidism is a silent epidemic creating symptoms that many physicians may not be able to link the absolute cause where in most cases, the cause may not be found within the thyroid itself. A weak immune system can often be the catalyst to an under-functioning thyroid; therefore, getting to the source of what is causing the immune system dysfunction can often revitalize the thyroid. Addressing dietary habits has been shown to support and heal hypothyroidism due to some foods showing a relationship with hypothyroidism. Specifically, those with low iodine intake have the potential to develop enlarged thyroids, called goiters, in addition to suffering from hypothyroidism. A well balanced diet with whole foods and recommended levels of vitamins and nutrients as well as cutting back on excessive sugars and fats.

Yoga practice supports the entire endocrine system, thus utilizing poses with sound vibration and repetition that compresses the throat has shown to improve functioning within the endocrine system. Breath traveling through the throat and feeling the constriction of breath within the throat flushes out held energy and serves as an energetic way to purify the throat chakra. Poses such as shoulder stand or bridge pose are especially stimulating for the thyroid gland. By accessing our innate resources we have more power in preventing and aid hormonal imbalances.

Self Healing Tools

Mind

Japa Meditation

Japa Meditation is an organized meditation where one focuses on a mantra or affirmation, such as "I am energized" or "I am peaceful." You may use any mantra that is fitting with your intention or circumstances. A mantra can be created based off of what you are asking for or what you need to find balance. It may be surrender, gratitude, creativity. Whatever the word or thought is, Japa Meditation connects you deeper to it.

Begin with sitting comfortably like you would for your regular meditation practice. Draw your attention to your breath allowing the natural flow of your breath to soften and relax you. Once you feel relaxed and present, begin to shift your attention from your breath to your mantra. Begin repeating your affirmation or mantra either in your head or verbally out loud. Continue gently repeating your intention. If you own a Mala you can use your Mala by holding each individual bead and repeating your intention to help keep you focused. As you continue, you may feel your mind begin to slip into a deeper meditative state. Whether you keep repeating the mantra or just simply be still with it - make this your mediation practice. Voicing it aloud stimulates the fifth chakra and can have a very positive effect in triggering a sense of wellness or feeling inspired.

Journaling

Journaling has the capacity to serve as a safe mental harbor. This practice touches both artistic and written expression allowing the writer to expunge mental congestion sourcing clarity, self affirmation, and emotional release. Similar to a caregiver having a special way of holding space for someone who is struggling, a blank page with an ink pen can support the patient by teaching them self regulation and self care. It is important to not only process our experiences, but also having the ability to express oneself. Having the means to mentally, emotionally, and spiritually to navigate our organic thought flow and experiences reconnects the mind with the present. This can also strengthen resiliency, stimulate neuroplasticity, and develop confidence.

Often, finding the words that accurately express how one feels can be challenging- or even daunting. But language often fails at exchanging shared meaning. It may even be through our withheld words that unleash chaos or unintentionally wounds another being. The ability for mankind to express and develop connection is magnified through each of our ability to connect within ourselves. This outer connection is reflected and influenced by our inner connection. It takes vulnerability and honesty to witness or observe the one looking back at us in the mirror. More often than not, the character traits we are so quick to criticize are the character traits within ourselves that we have an aversion towards.

Journaling can serve as a way to explore the inward collection of thoughts, fears, and feelings without responding with a compulsive reaction. Journaling creates space between our emotions and our actions thus helping the writer connect deeper with themselves and soothe the reactive fuse that could lead to destructive behaviors. It also gives insight to the writer regarding habitual thought forms and patterns that could invite one to reconstruct his or her daily routines and habits in healthy, supportive ways. Writing has been connected to relieving stress and cultivating resolution. By starting a journal one evokes a new lens on self transformation to document experiences and process challenges that naturally emerge in life. Let this space empower your voice, chisel your truths, and evaporate the thoughts and feelings that no longer serve you.

Body

See Yoga Glossary for Fifth Chakra Poses

Vocalizing Your Soul

Different lineages of yoga implement vocals into practice. For example, Kirtan comes from the lineage of Bhakti Yoga which refers to the yoga of devotion. This practice involves utilizing the vibrations of sound through chanting and activating different parts of the body. The tone of our voice alone navigates along the chakra continuum. As our voice goes higher, we can feel the vibration all the way up to our forehead. As our voice gets lower, we can feel the vibration from the sound in our belly. The dial tone of our voice impacts the way we may feel when we sing or chant.

A branch of therapeutic yoga known as Phoenix Rising Yoga Therapy implements the use of dialogue to support the student in taking inquiry of the present moment and experiences during the practice. The sessions often occur in a one on one setting where the facilitator utilizes assisted yoga postures, dialogue, and mindfulness to cultivate a process that is client-centered and non-directive. As the teacher takes the student to his or her edge, the use of dialogue encourages the student to verbally express his or her experience. The edge is the volume dial of intensity in a pose. Often the edge we choose on the mat reflects the edge we choose in our life, however, the intention is to learn to live in harmony with our edges exploring that edge without fear but presence.

Another type of yoga that utilizes vocals is Kripalu. An introspective type of practice, Kripalu puts emphasis on learning from the body. It begins with noticing the unique experience in each pose and then slowly introducing more challenging poses holding them longer. Some poses and sequences combined with "shhhh" on the exhale or "mmmmm" on the exhale invite the student to explore the sensation that occur in the body when the breath moves with voice. Often it is used as a tool for personal growth and self empowerment teaching one to tap into their own innate wisdom and inner resources rather than being dependent upon external guidances. Each sensation is greeted with tenderness and each practice is approached with an attitude of prayer since Kripalu treats the body as the temple.

There are many other ways to implement sound into the yoga practice through creative expression, singing, sighing, and simply talking; each has the potential to strengthen the vocal cords and larynx. By knowing the blueprint of the chakras, one can infuse the deficient chakra with sound which actives the glands through pressure and vibration to restore energy and wellness. Sound is derived from the diaphragm to power the larynx, but many people exhaust the throat which can create tenderness, pain, and energetic blocks. Through practice and mindfulness, the physical manifestation of voice begins to strengthen along with clarity in words, truth, and the courage to speak.

Although research is still underway, there have been studies conducted to measure the health benefits of singing and participating in choir. An exploratory study at a university college choral society expressed that 84% of the participants shared that singing improved their health in some way, such as lung function, socially, stress management, and over all improvement of mood. Other studies showed participants reporting feelings of positivity and relaxation after singing. Much like observing one's breath, singing can be implemented into one's practice and life to support wellness and restore the chakras.

Breath

Jalandhara Bandha

The Bandas are energetic locks or contractive energy that hold energy into a central location of the body. Jalandhara Bandha engages and tones the throat muscles while energizing the fifth chakra. One can implement deep, slow breathing with this Bandha along with utilizing it in his or her yoga practice.

To begin, find your way into a comfortable seated position with palms facing down onto the knees. Take a deep breath in, and sigh it out clearing any stale energy contained within the spine. Begin to slowly inhale to two thirds of your lung's breath capacity and hold the breath dropping the chin down towards the chest drawing it in so the back of neck stays long and does not round. To deepen the throat lock, allow the shoulders to roll forward. Hold this for as long as it is comfortable and without forcing or straining. When you are ready to release, slowly bring the chin up and take a breath in through the nose and let it out. Allow the breath to return to your natural rhythm and pace. The throat lock is contraindicated for heart disease and high blood pressure. With practice, Jalandhara Bandha has been shown to improve circulation and breath capacity along with balancing metabolism in the thyroid.

THIRD EYE CHAKRA

The Gem of Mentality

**"The soul becomes dyed with the color
of its thoughts." - Marcus Aurelius**

The sixth chakra, also known as the "Third Eye" chakra, is located in the space between the eyebrows. The sixth chakra is associated with the hypothalamus and pituitary glands where the executive functioning of the brain occurs. Ajna is the Sanskrit word for command. This chakra is responsible for the command center of our minds cultivating intuition, thinking symbolically, awareness, clarity, and wisdom. This chakra supports the development of our personal identity and our ability to perceive patterns in the world. This is the space that holds one's capacity to be mindful and intuitive, making constructive decisions based on supportive, strong notions. Meditation, mindfulness, self-reflection, education, and the witnessing mind (paying attention to external and internal activity with detached awareness) are some of the different ways to activate this chakra. Causes of imbalance include disappointment, reluctance to make an effort, having no joy for the future, ignoring truth, insensitivity, poor memory, difficulty visualizing, delusions, self- victimizing, anxiety, depression, and denial.

Perception plays a large role in this chakra and its imbalances. Therefore, whether it's facing suffering or an illusion, choosing to seek truth or healing induces balance and yields wisdom. The genesis of wisdom is pain and the sixth chakra is the final product of what was experienced in the first and second chakras. With this chakra comes the realization and practice that each person has an innate ability to connect with peace and that the entrance is found within the mind and through body. Ultimately, it is free will that governs one's capacity to experience this. If deep serenity resonates in nature, then deep serenity naturally is found within us. It just takes creating stillness for serene discovery.

Meditation

"Mediation is really a non-doing. It is the only human endeavor I know of that does not involve trying to get somewhere else but, rather, emphasizes being where you already are." (p.55) John Kabat-Zinn, Full Catastrophe Living

Mediation is simply just being. It is the art of falling into the space between each thought. I teach meditation to my students by having them begin in a comfortable seat. If the participant is forcing themselves to sit up straight, then they are contradicting the whole purpose of surrender and being. Therefore, do not force an 'ideal' postural position, but be comfortable. Mediation can even be practiced while lying down. However, if one chooses to lie down for meditation, be mindful of not falling asleep. Often I will guide my students to witness the sensations within their bodies, noticing how the breath oscillates with the rhythm and flow of the body, and maybe drawing their awareness to their pulse within their hands, feet, or face. This practice is simply a non-doing, a channel to relax with detached awareness and be still.

Much of our time is spent judging, directing, fixing, or doing something- even if we aren't physically doing these things the mind fixates on productivity or being occupied by external stimuli. Meditation is an opportunity to tune into yourself and experience you. We hardly attend to the awareness of our own mind and how much that drives us. And for many people, the thought of being alone with their mind may be terrifying. This is because we have been so conditioned to preoccupy ourselves due to living in such a plugged in culture, that just being with the fruitfulness of our own mind may take time to get comfortable with. However, when we slow down to smell the bouquet of flowers sitting on the counter, to feel warmth on our fingertips from the cup of hot tea and how that sensation travels through the hand- these details nourish our ability to truly show up for life. To be present without expectation, while savoring each moment and tribulation, contributes to building a quality infused life. When we fill ourselves up from the inside, serving becomes easier and we become better. This is the essence of mindfulness. Meditation provokes us to touch base with what lies beneath the story, beneath the circumstances, beneath our tribulations.

Burnout is generated by our inability to slow down causing us to 'over do.' In Mindfulness Based Stress Reduction, they teach the saying "You are a human being, not a human doing." The phrase identifies that we must take time to remind ourselves of who we are and hold space for self-care. Meditation leads one to a new level of knowing - instilling patience, clarity, and a focused mind. Slowing down is the fastest way to efficiency. When we care for ourselves and take time to rest; the nervous system will return to balance, immunity goes up, and our ability to retain information improves. Here are a few reasons to begin meditating.

The left prefrontal cortex of the brain gets larger when we meditate. This means that our ability to make wise decisions becomes heightened, affect regularity is balanced, we feel more purpose, stronger capability in combating depression (yes, meditation cultivates happiness), we have clarity in seeing the bigger picture, improves mood, and other physiological benefits.

Also, research has shown that a larger prefrontal cortex can correlate with a living a longer life.

Improves sleep. Meditation and Yoga Nidra stimulate lactic acid removal and muscle relaxation creating deeper sleep. Meditation also enhances melatonin levels by augmenting the synthesis in the pineal gland. As one continues to practice meditation, it strengthens the body's ability to consciously relax itself to achieve restfulness and better quality of sleep. Meditation is also a means of ventilation, in other words, meditation helps flush out the stressful events of the day and move into bedtime with peace and tender relaxation.

Meditation induces neuroplasticity, or the brain's ability to change in response to life experiences by creating new neural pathways. This allows the neurons within the brain to counterbalance the effects of injury, trauma, and cognitive dysfunction by creating new responses to one's environment and circumstances. Recent studies have shown that neuroplasticity is a substantial way of dealing with trauma opening a new capacity of healing through practices such as meditation, intentional dialogue, breathing, and yoga.

Improves immunity and initiates vagal toning. Deep breathing in general increases lymph flow within the body. It is important for our immune system functioning that the lymph flows properly through the body. Furthermore, chronic stress weakens the immune system due to the body being flooded with hormones such as epinephrine and cortisol. Overtime, the hypothalamic-pituitary-adrenal axis response within the body will suppress the immune system which could lead to disease and illness within the body creating low vagal tone. The vagus nerve is highly responsible for collecting information within the body and sending it to the brain for the brain to process. When there is dysfunction here, it impacts the entire body's ability to function properly. Our ability to check into the body (through mediums such as mindfulness or body awareness) and see how we are feeling comes from the vagus nerve. The vagus nerve supplies parasympathetic fibers to almost all of our internal organs which also impacts our ability to self regulate. Meditation, or practices where our interception is activated, stimulates vagal toning and strengthens our parasympathetic response within the body turning the limbic system back on so the executive functioning of our bodies can regulate and manage stress in a healthy way.

Improves Heart Rate Variability. Heart Rate Variability is a way to measure the effects of stress on the heart and within the body. Research has shown that the slow breathing technique used in meditation has reported significant improvement in balancing the nervous system by increasing parasympathetic activity and reflecting higher HRV. Meditation cultivates greater resilience to stress supported by biofeedback, which has shown meditation practices such as slow breathing and conscious relaxation improves heart rate variability.

A recent Harvard study showed that *meditating for half an hour a day actually caused changes in the brain's structure* noticing a primary difference in the posterior cingulate which influences how our mind wanders. The study showed changes inn the left hippocampus assisting in cognition, learning, emotion regulation, and memory. Also within the temporo parietal junction which influences the interpretation of our experiences, compassion, and empathy. Neurotransmitters are also positively influenced along with the amygdala which regulates our stress response.

Meditation is leverage to experiencing oneself as is in that moment. Once the individual lets go of striving for results, but focuses carefully on whatever experiences are present, while accepting things as they are- one may achieve deep peace through meditation. Sometimes uncomfortable feelings may arise, however, practicing witnessing those feeling; not identify or explaining what they are but just attending the experience. A wonderful exercise to try if this happens is to separate the experience from the emotion and to simply feel the emotion. For example, the feeling of anger because somebody manipulated you into doing something you are not proud of. Let go of what the source of that anger is. Feel angry. Now, couple that anger with love. In other words, all of our emotions are an extension of love. We hurt because we love, we are excited because we love, we fight because we love, we are disappointed because we love, we cry because we love so on and so forth. Anger is the shadow of the heart- so coupling that with love. I am angry because I love. Now practice softening the face and the body as you feel angry and feel the anger dissipate slowly. As the ancient Chinese proverb goes- "love made a body." Notice, witness, and let it go. There is an unfolding, there is an unwinding. When we sever the identity of circumstances and emotions to be who we are beneath those stories- we find not only healing but begin to realize that we are the source of our own peace.

MINDFULNESS

Mindfulness is a basic human function of paying attention to the present moment in a non-judging way. Research has shown that as one deepens their connection with moment-to-moment awareness, it expands the capacity for optimum living and dealing with stress more effectively. Mindfulness can be developed through meditation practices or by slowing down to pay more attention with what is unfolding within the present moment, and overtime becomes more habitual in lifestyle and thought patterns. The way one perceives his or her experiences influences the reaction to those experiences. Mindfulness supports one into being less reactive and effectively responding to the present moment need. There has been an abundance of scientific research on mindfulness demonstrating that the mechanisms of mindfulness produce not only relaxation, but also prominent shifts in cognition, emotions, and behavior that work collaboratively to improve health. Research is also beginning to prove that attitudes of compassion, acceptance, and greater attention refines self-awareness and facilitates resilience which can help relieve one from suffering generating optimal health and wellbeing.

Mindfulness has an amazing capacity to teach self-compassion. Self-compassion is our ability to meet ourselves where we are in whatever moment arises. By having an attitude of self-compassion, one can effectively respond to what they need rather than shaming or becoming frustrated with themselves. The compassion we offer to ourselves is the foundation to what we hold for others. This is the practice of treating ourselves with the same kindness we would for a friend or someone we love. Making this a habit begins to fill the "longing" or the "hole" that can often divert us from peace. Using mindfulness to cultivate self-compassion would be practicing a shift in attitude. For instance, if you look into the mirror and immediately become critical about your face using mindfulness would say "Oh, I see that I am being critical of myself, I see I do not like this about myself." It begins with witnessing the behavior and then shifting the thought platform to self-kindness. It is shifting from viewing abnormalities and differences into common humanity. To be human is to be imperfect, so practicing self-compassion grounds one deeper into the relationship and being with whatever the present moment is. Gratitude is also a great practice to produce abundance and self-compassion.

Whether through loving-kindness meditations or being present, mindfulness invites one to participate completely in the present moment with whatever is- not identified by the current challenges or circumstances but by living inspired (especially because these things and all things are temporary) and engaging the experience as an opportunity to be refined into a better version of you.

Saying no is a form of self-compassion. When we overexert ourselves our immune system depletes making us vulnerable to illness and sunder from presence. There must always be a balance in what we give and when we give we give with containment. Self-compassion heightens our aptitude in combating stress and grounding to unearth relaxation and restoration. It is okay to say no. Saying no is one of the most powerful acts of self care one can practice because it helps us preserve our energy and our health. Practicing self-love and compassion assists in developing a meaningful relationship with ourselves and latently inspires others to do the same.

Loving-Kindness Meditation

This form of meditation creates a foundation of friendliness, kindness, and compassion drawing out the basic goodness in others or yourself. The method is phrase-based or through visualizations. The practice below is the phrase-based method. You may also create your own phrases with the intention to direct and receive feelings of kindness and compassion. If the mind wanders, just bring it back to the phrases. You may sit comfortably or relax on your back. The techniques are the same as traditional meditation instructions.

Towards yourself:

So often love is defined as an outward reflection of adoration towards someone or something, however, when we return to the source of love it always leads us back within. The Golden Rule, "love your neighbor as you love yourself" exemplifies that self-love is the foundation upon which we love others. For we can only extend to others what we have offered ourselves so setting an intention to reconnect with loving-kindness for yourself may enhance your ability to show up for others and for yourself.

This meditation offers a way to counter negative, critical feelings we may cultivate towards ourselves. We must acknowledge that sometimes it is not easy to love ourselves because we are constantly immersed in comparing and striving towards outward accomplishments that have no relationship with who we are at our essence. These things are illusions that distract us from our ability to source abundance from within- to feel whole. We are so obsessed with searching for happiness that we forget to happily seek. This is the art of being present.

- May I be happy
- May I be healthy

- May I be peaceful
- May I be safe

Repeating these phrases to yourself feeling each wish vividly and as genuine as you can towards yourself. If you feel nothing for yourself, it doesn't mean you are doing it wrong but you are simply planting seeds by your intention.

Towards others:

Loving-Kindness takes the practitioner through a variety of different roles that individuals may play a part of in your life. The first, as we went over is yourself. The following are as followed.

- A teacher or mentor
- Loved one (family or friend)
- Neutral person (this may be somebody you saw at the grocery store or a neighbor you may not really know)
- Difficult person (someone who may be defiant or challenging in your life)
- All people

You can repeat the same style of phrases as you did for yourself or even create new ones such as "Let him/her live with peace," "Let him/her feel safe and protected," etc.

Loving-Kindness meditation is a method of prayer for the goodwill of others and a way to harvest more understanding to others or even the ability to release destructive habits of anger or hate towards the difficult person. This practice towards yourself can help you stand firm in who you are, especially when dealing with difficult people. Loving-kindness does not mean being a doormat; it prepares you to ground in your own wisdom and truth with the clarity to be assertive if needed. Mindfulness can draw the strength to not take personally what difficult people may say, but understanding that hurt people hurt people and it is their suffering that is causing them to project their shadow onto you.

And if this happens, offering loving-kindness and compassion for yourself and the situation.

Because mindfulness redirects one to the present moment, it produces better task performing throughout the day including a broadened intellectual capacity, problem solving, acquisition of skills, and a more fulfilling outlook on life. Mindfulness may look like pausing for a few moments to feel or pay attention to breath or even chewing your food slower to taste the details of the details. It is slow. It is watchful. It is mindful. If a stressful event occurs the path of responding isn't negative, driven by reactive emotions. The path of responding is informed by emotions, mediated by awareness, and producing clear communication with self-care rather than dysfunctional behavior patterns. We must be aware how our reactivity can create deeper problems within our lives.

"Know this, my beloved brothers: let every person be quick to hear, slow to speak, slow to anger;" James 1:19

It is normal for the mind to wander, so if your mind wanders it doesn't mean you are doing it wrong. It is an opportunity to notice that your mind is wandering and then bring it back to the present through breath, sensation, or intention. It is a process and a practice, therefore, if any thoughts arise such as "I am doing this wrong" pause and bring it back to the present. That is mindfulness; to derail cluttered thought platforms and ground the mind into the unfolding moment before you. Like meditation, it is a non-striving. Mindfulness is being.

Body Scans

Body scanning invites you to fully experience your body in that present moment. These are very useful for chronic pain, insomnia, anxiety, and improving body awareness. A body scan is an active process of sensory awareness moving through each part of the body. When practicing, it is important to utilize detached awareness only, which is a way to witness the sensation within the specified body part but not reacting or becoming involved with that part of the body. Body scans are slow with methodical attention and a "non-striving" type of listening to the body. Some practices move from the feet to the top of the head, where others may move in a specified pattern.

Practice:

Lying down in a comfortable position, begin to take a deep breath in. Sigh it out. Draw your awareness down to your feet. Begin to squeeze and engage the muscles within the feet. Squeeze the feet and exhale relax your feet. Let it go.

Draw your awareness down to your calf muscles. Begin to squeeze and engage your calf muscles. Squeeze and exhale relax your calves. Let it go.

Draw your awareness into your thighs. The hamstrings, quads, the entire thigh. Begin to squeeze and engage the muscles within the thigh. Hold and exhale. Let it go.

Draw your awareness into your buttocks, hips, and pelvic floor. Squeeze the buttocks, engage the pelvic floor. Squeeze the entire pelvic region and exhale. Let it go.

Draw your awareness into the belly. Begin to engage your core and tightening the muscles within your abdomen. Squeeze and exhale, let it go.

Draw your awareness into your chest. The heart space, thoracic region. Begin to squeeze engaging the chest muscles. Exhale. Let it go.

Draw your awareness down through your arms into your hands. Begin to bring your hands into fist squeezing and engaging the muscles all through your arms, hands balled into fist. Squeeze and exhale relax your hands and arms. Let it go.

Draw your awareness into your shoulders and upper arms. Engage and squeeze the shoulders, tightening into the upper back and arms. Exhale relax your body. Let it go.

Draw your awareness into your neck. Begin to squeeze and constricting the throat and maybe your chin makes a silly face. Squeeze and let it go.

Finally, draw your awareness into your face. Begin to squeeze the face making silly faces squeezing. And exhale relax your face. Let it go.

Feel the whole body relax, softening here. Eyes closed. Take a deep breath in. And sigh it out.

Breath Awareness in Mindfulness

Feelings come and go like clouds in a windy sky. Conscious breathing is my anchor. ~Thích Nhất Hạnh

Breathing itself is essential to our wellbeing. It is the deepest expression of our vitality and is that which connects the mind to body. Breathing affects the body on not only a physiological level, but also our psychology. The breath is a huge catalyst to how we feel and affects the nervous system. Slow exhales cool the nervous system stimulating our parasympathetic response. This is why when one is having an anxiety attack; the first thing the therapist or caregiver responds with is getting the individual to return to their breath. Slow exhale, deep breathing. Inhales have been shown to have an energizing effect within the body. For example, during an anxiety attack one's breath may be rapid and short causing an arousal within the sympathetic nervous system.

The breath can serve as a guide to bring us back to the present moment. It enhances our awareness to what is going on inside the body as we tune into the sensations surfacing in that moment. When an individual pauses to check in with his or her breath, it becomes the catalyst to experience existence on a subtle level inviting one to slow down. Mindfulness and meditation utilize the breath as though it anchors us into ourselves allowing us to drop down into the body and feel, thus creating the foundation for clarity.

The yoga practice uses these principles to influence the experience in each pose. Energizing classes may utilize more quick inhales, were a restorative class may encourage slow, long exhales. Breathing has mood-altering effects and stimulates hormones such as prolactin, oxytocin, and dopamine. Controlled breathing itself moves lymph, improves heart rate variability, can lower blood pressure, and deactivates a hyper aroused nervous system. When we don't breath properly, less oxygen gets to the brain derailing proper functioning and can instill feelings of anxiety or irritation. Breath awareness begins with noticing your natural breath and how it exists within your body. Whether used as a tool in mindfulness, meditation, or the yoga practice- the breath is the ultimate source of energy and awareness.

Walking Meditation

Walking meditation is simply paying close attention to the sensations you feel, such as your foot planting down onto the ground and then lifting it and so on. It is also paying close attention to what thoughts arise as you walk. It invites one to hold a deeper awareness of inner listening. Where to walk, when to stop, where to sit and pause, or where to go. It is a form of listening to the wisdom of intuitive direction and the process of feeling the details of each experience.

Insomnia

Fifty to seventy million Americans have a sleep disorder of some sort and most sleep disorders are caused by chronic pain, fatigue, stress, or anxiety. As we know, lack of sleep depletes the immune system and causes stress. Sleep disorders can generate a vicious cycle of frustration and pain driving one to resort to sleep medications or supplement use. When we use outside resources to medicate a sleep disorder it may lead to dependency and the body may no longer produce the proper amount of chemicals and hormones to induce sleep naturally. Furthermore, seeking sleep aids may not necessarily correct the root problem to why one is suffering from insomnia.

Holistic interventions can help redirect the patient back into self-sustainability and address the underlying causes for the sleep disorder. For instance, if one deals with an anxiety disorder, the nervous system is over-activated, which hinders the body's ability to relax sufficiently in order to fall or stay asleep. Yoga, meditation, and lifestyle choices not only help with sleep, but has shown with evidence based research that they soothe the nervous system back into optimal functioning building resilience to triggers and stress. More often than not, insomnia is a result of an underlying problem such as environmental, life style choices, social, illnesses, or mental activity that may prevent restful sleep. It is imperative to identify the source of imbalance in order for the patient to implement constructive lifestyle changes.

This begins by identifying what type of insomnia one is suffering from. Primary Insomnia is associated with life changes, stress, emotional, imbalanced schedules, and dysfunctional habits whereas secondary insomnia is the product of a specific medical condition and/or medication. For example, secondary insomnia may be associated with cardiovascular problems such as high blood pressure, nervous system hyperarousal such as inflammation in the body, obesity, body pain, overactive thyroid, menopause, or respiratory problems. Therefore, identifying what is causing the insomnia will exemplify where to begin in addressing the sleep disorder.

Self Care for Insomnia

Yogic practices and mindfulness with consistency can play a key role in healing a sleep disorder. Reducing muscle tension and muscle cramps, yoga improves heart rate variability and soothes a hyperactive nervous system. See benefits of meditation. Furthermore, meditation clears the mind and invites an attitude of acceptance and non-striving. A mistake people often make is to strive for sleep, trying to fall asleep. But when we 'try' to sleep it becomes an active process. Therefore, practicing relaxing and mindfulness may induce sleep much quicker and promote restfulness rather than a frustrated attempt to try and force sleep.

Though it seems contradictory, it is common to be too tired to sleep. Restorative yoga is a productive way to relax the muscles and stimulate the parasympathetic nervous system. In restorative yoga, the patient would use props such as pillows, bolsters, blankets, or blocks to adjust the body into a supportive stretch that allows the body to open while the patient relaxes into the pose. Each pose is held between three to ten minutes. See yoga pose glossary for further examples.

Block Occipital Massage
(Great for Neck Discomfort)

At the base of the skull resides the suboccipital muscles. When massaged and stimulated, it shifts the nervous system into a relaxed state. Take a block to the middle level setting it onto the ground. Then rest that bone that protrudes at the base of skull onto the edge of the block. Once stabilized, begin to gently rock the head side to side and feel the massage at the base of skull. Close the eyes and breath as you intuitively let the head rock side to side at your own pace. Remember to breathe in through the nose and out the nose. Avoid this if there are any cervical herniation of the disc, recent neck surgeries, or if it feels uncomfortable.

Even if you are lying in bed, you can place a bolster or blanket beneath the knees to help support the low back. Restorative yoga is especially nice to do in the evening before you go to bed to prepare the body for relaxation. Focusing on your breath, prayer, body awareness, or intention helps redirect the mind into the present moment to prepare for sleep. A well-rounded yoga practice, or simply deep stretching the body throughout the day keeps the muscles open and improves the ability to consciously relax. Yoga Nidra is a fruitful relaxation technique to do before bed to relax both the mind and body. Yoga Nidra and Meditation have been shown to be more restful than sleep itself yielding more benefits such as releasing tense muscles, pain management, the job of full recovery within the nervous system and reviving the mind, thus improving the quality of sleep. These holistic techniques equip you with self-sustainable methods to deliberately control your ability to relax and achieve rest.

Breathing for Insomnia

"Breath is the finest gift of nature. Be grateful for this wonderful gift." - Amit Ray

Below are a few breathing techniques to help with sleep:

Breathing Ratios

Inhale through the nose for four counts, hold at the top for seven counts, and exhale out the nose for eight counts. Repeat.

Inhale through the nose for three counts, and exhale out the nose for six counts.

Sighing it out is a good way to release built up tension in the body. Inhale for three counts, hold at the top, and big sigh out the mouth.

Ujjayi breath

Translated to Victorious Breathing, this breathing exercise calms the mind improving concentration, regulates heating within the body, diminishes pain from headaches, helps to relieve sinus pressure, decreases phlegm, and strengthens the nervous and digestive systems.

To begin, the patient must constrict the back of the throat to make the breath audible like the sound of the ocean or sounding like Darth Vader breathing. The ujjayi breath flows in and out of the nose and the constriction in the back of the throat is the same you would make if you were going to whisper or to say "ha" (but with lips closed). Practice a few rounds and the way I recommend to my students is you know you are doing it right when it sounds like the ocean is drawing upon the shoreline and being pulled back out to sea. The sound itself can be very meditative and soothing while catering to our ability to relax within the body.
How to:

Sit in a comfortable position with your spine upright and your eyes closed.

Inhale slowly through the nose and as you exhale out the mouth produce the sound "HHHAAAA."

Now, inhale again through the nose and on your exhale keep the mouth closed maintaining the same position as your throat did with the "HHAA." The exhale is "HHAA" with the mouth closed.

On your inhales, maintain same throat position as your exhaling-feeling the breath brush against the roof of your mouth.

Make sure the sound originates from your throat. It should sound almost like darth vader breathing or ocean waves.

Continue this. You can also do this breath lying down.

There is an enchantment when one is connected with the breath gaining new inner resources to consciously source his or her own peace. Whether it is the process of falling asleep or feelings of being overwhelmed, return to your breath. Let the breath bring you back home to your body. It is essential to 'let the breath breathe you' when you are trying to fall asleep- witness the breath. Feel where it navigates within the body and soon it turns into a form of meditation.

Mindfulness for Insomnia

Influencing the mind will liberate the mind. Mindfulness for insomnia begins with self-compassion and instilling life style changes to help slow the circadian rhythm within the body. After dinner beginning to talk slower, walk slower, and other ways to create a slower rhythm encouraging gentleness and rest to prepare for sleep. Mindfulness can encourage one to withdraw his or her senses in order to turn inward- bringing your practice to bed. Being mindful of the environment where you are sleeping.

Is the environment calm and quiet? Does the environment feel safe and relaxing? What kind of light are you exposed to? The hypothalamus is stimulated by light. Light decreases melatonin and may be the reason why it is hard to fall asleep, or why you may wake up in the middle of the night. Is the environment too hot or are you too cold? So be mindful and aware of your environment since these things may play a key role in perpetuating a sleep disorder.

Another factor that may influence a sleep disorder is one's nightly routine. What we do during the day ventilates what we don't have to bring to bed, so maybe using dinnertime as the space to discuss to details of the day, frustrations, and plans for tomorrow. Using the evening as time for self-care practices may help deactivate the nervous system shifting it into relaxation mode. Slowing down.

A consistent bedtime is also very helpful for producing quality sleep along with not eating right before you go to bed. Be mindful of your medication and its effects on sleep because that is a common reason people may have sleep disorders. Essentially, the choices you make before you go to bed can deeply influence how you sleep or the unhealthy habits that may arise from inconsistency, stimulation, and stress evoked within the evening.

Self Healing Tools

Palming

Begin by rubbing your hands together to create warmth. Once the hands feel warm close your eyes and take your palms against the eyelids. Feel the warmth and sensation from the hands. Take a deep breath in, feeling the inhale expand into the forehead. And then flush a big sigh out the mouth. And then be here for a few moments feeling the natural breath flowing in and out of the body.

BODY

See Yoga Glossary for Sixth Chakra Poses

CROWN CHAKRA

Awakening to Wellness

"It is useless to seek yourself outside yourself."

The crown chakra is the seventh of the chakras and is associated with the pineal gland, which deals with the mind's interpretation of night and day and is also associated with the gap junction cells in the skull. Sahassrara is the Sanskrit word for thousandfold which implies the infinite nature of this chakra. Like the sixth chakra, the crown's nature is around thought, meaning, and awakening. Extended bliss and peace are the characteristics associated along with no physical element present based solely in spiritual and philosophical concepts. In order to live in mindfulness and well-being the support of the lower chakras are imperative for this last chakra to reign. This space symbolizes the highest state of enlightenment and spiritual development. As the lower chakras display life and relationship development the upper chakras are wisdom, intellect, and spiritual development. Mental health imbalances are often due to patterns in perception, however, by participating in exercising the mind and mentality one can support their mental ailments. The crown chakra is much more about awakening than healing. Awakening happens through the ability to develop our capacity of stillness, witnessing, and non attachment. Non Attachment comes from the ability to release expectation being open to whatever the moment brings. Expectation can serve as the thief of love leading to disappointment and resentfulness. Honing into the fact that this life is temporary gives us the peace of knowing that nothing is actually guaranteed. It takes practice and concentration to embed these into our being, but over time and even with acknowledgement we can generate peace in our lives through our attitudes with each experience.

Making Meaning

In my experience of coaching hundreds of clients, a common question I ask is, "What is your heartfelt hope for yourself and for your life?" Every single person's reply embodies the hope of making an impact or living in a way that contributes to the collective. From familial to global, people desire to create meaning out of their lives. The seventh chakra is about the realization of that meaning. The right to know one's dharma or purpose in life. This is never fully realized by the individual as our lives continuously evolve as we age, but through each moment we create a collection of pieces that reflect what our lives mean. These meaningful experiences become a positive constellation of results that contribute to our overall sense of purpose.

As the seventh chakra is fortified by information, our meaning is constructed by interactions and the relationship to experiences within our lives. Our relationship to our experiences and even lack thereof correlate to whether or not we feel fulfilled. Because life happens through us, the container in which we hold and interpret our experiences generate the meaning we make from them. When one reflects on the turning points in their life that have shaped them into who they are today, the stories told are those of deep transformational experiences they've cultivated even deeper meaning with whether sourced from trauma or enlightenment.

Meaning created begins to form the structure of which we live in accordance to establishing our moral framework and purpose behind each choice we make.

Because we are a species of categorizing and interpreting, meaning comes from our hope to create a deeper understanding to why things happen the way they do or to source a justifiable explanation for an event witnessed or experienced. Thus resulting to us holding boundaries or living by morals that expound the meaning affiliated. When we live in accordance we may feel secure, fulfilled, and satisfied however when we act in violation to our conscience in may lead to feelings of guilt or shame. Through forgiveness, compassion, and letting go we can move back into our personal standards as we continue to evolve into a better, healed version of ourselves.

Meaning made can be shared through stories and council to others. We take strength from one another's stories. Shared meaning passes healing and inspiration onto others that they may move forward through the obstacles, challenges, and/or frustrations that naturally occur within life. I believe deeply that our experiences qualify us in so many ways because everything you go through, grows you. Each of us hold a unique story, lesson, and significance, yet our vulnerability in sharing draws us closer and creates communities where people can feel supported in their life. Many imbalances or illnesses can be stripped down exposing that the source was caused by not feeling supported or not feeling loved. When we have the courage to be vulnerable and be human, others can relate and healing persists. Even more so, growth persists. New information is collected into understanding being alchemized into wisdom. Wisdom is healed pain and wise men seek council. A people who share meaning, collaborate, and support one another generates abundance into this life and this world.

We sabotage ourselves when we disengage from one another and form competitive initiatives collapsing into our own egos. Deepak Chopra defines ego as Edging God Out. Feeding the ego creates selfish motives that separates us from abundance launching us into feelings of inadequacy and lack. We become hungry for validation and begin to behave in spite, fear, and solitary. When we forsake others we forsake ourselves. Buying into the ego and living from a place of scarcity clouds our ability to draw meaning throwing the chakra modality off balance.

Apathy is the shadow of meaning. Apathy may be used to further justify stagnation and reject accountability. The truth is, no one can make some care, the individual must decide on their own. I have witnessed many people drain themselves and become abused by another's indifference. Addicts are more likely to relapse when they are forced by a loved one to get treatment. Veterans suffering from depression and PTSD are likely not to implement therapies when forced by a loved one to get treatment. Patients suffering from heart problems due to obesity are less likely to make critical lifestyle changes when forced by a loved one to get treatment. Authentic, sustainable change is a by product of the individual motivated by personal conviction and then directly seeking change.

However, this is usually prompted by providence or an event that softens the shell apathy has solidified. In dealing with someone who demonstrates apathy, to maintain self care one must react with compassion and surrender. More often than not, the real culprit of apathy is derived from lower body chakra imbalances and blocks that have not yet been addressed. Making meaning of the relationship with the apathetic individual serves as curriculum to be refined into compassion and moving forward in your own growth and optimum living.

As the saying goes, when the student is ready the teacher comes. To maintain a balanced seventh chakra, living inspired by these things are vital to spiritual development and connection. Invite the shorelines of your mind to expand into a deeper capacity for meaning and understanding, thus yielding growth and quality from each experience that surfaces with each day.

Prayer

Prayer is a platform for intention. Through prayer we actively knit ourselves into the tapestry of providence and align our thinking with love, with hope, and with compassion infusing the present moment with an open and humble heart. It creates the space to show up for life. Whether it be the ideas and hopes collected from the realms of consciousness or simply having dialogue with God; prayer ventilates the mind from fears and anxieties that even though at the present moment may not have an answer there is promise of growth, change, and transformation granted through providence. Prayer is a way to surface the murmurings of the heart and connecting that to something greater.

Prayer invites one to go deeper into stillness replacing anxious thoughts with peaceful thoughts and directing the nervous system back into harmony. Through prayer and meditation we begin to align our thinking to God's thinking- infinite, love, and surrender. There is no magic method for how to pray; it is your intimate connection to Spirit.

I often encourage my students to begin their meditation practice with prayer and then turn inward for listening facilitating a way to surrender any mental hindrances, worries, or distractions to God. The chakras began because the Vedic people wanted to return to God. There is a physiological healing by expanding the mind through prayer and meditation. Let yourself return to your beloved.

Self Healing Tools

Yoga Nidra

Throughout this book I hope you have begun to understand the power of our subconscious mind and how it far exceeds the conscious mind in terms of impacting the physical body and default behaviors. Yoga Nidra is a powerful way to access the subconscious mind initiating many benefits in healing the underlying causes to many ailments. Many researchers claim that our conscious mind operates at only 3-15% of its capability, however, mindfulness techniques such as yoga nidra expand our conscious mind yielding many positive results such as those already expressed in meditation and other neurological, physiological, and spiritual benefits.

Because meditation induces complete relaxation in the mind and body, many claim that yoga nidra is even more relaxing than sleep. In fact, yoga nidra is far better than sleep for releasing tense muscles, pain management, and transitioning the mind and body quickly from stress to calm. Yoga Nidra teaches conscious control of relaxation and compliments sleep in completing the job of full recovery within the nervous system and reviving the mind. Many practitioners find that yoga nidra improves their quality of sleep drastically.

The practice can be used to shape the mind and alter our approach to life increasing resilience to help combat stress, depression and anxiety. The mind is able to think clearly and retain information better and is believed to improve concentration and memory. It provides a new platform of thinking allowing us to find a place of inner recourse utilizing positive thought forms to shift negative mental thought forms that may be reinforcing unhealthy lifestyle choices or pain. Based on our life experiences, we often tag additional meaning to our thoughts and the stories behind them. "I thought" is a genetically engineered perception that is constructed by an individual's empirical meaning. Yoga Nidra utilizes the subconscious to shred previous beliefs tied to emotions or sensations by pervading the 'thought' with present moment details of being whole and separate from the fabricated perceptions. This occurs by accessing the "witnessing" mind cultivating more space between our emotions and our reactions, our ability to detach from toxic identities and thoughts, and welcoming the present moment authentically.

Although Yoga Nidra is a great way to bring the whole body back into balance, it correlates greatly with the seventh chakra because it relates to spiritual growth and development. Yoga Nidra holds the capacity to tap into a greater knowing of purpose and heightening our physiology to attain what we want to achieve in the quadrants of our life. The physical benefits are stated and supported by science, however, measuring the psychological and spiritual benefits of the practice have been expounded through what many practitioners have experienced themselves. The unification between science and this ancient practice delineate why neurology shows increased brain function and how it has produced these fulfilling emotional and lifestyle choices made by those who have used yoga nidra as an outlet for healing.

Furthermore, because Yoga Nidra acknowledges what is right with the participant (in other words, it focuses on wholeness first), the participant can disassociate from dysfunctional identities or the attachment to pain and work through affirmative and functional components of his or her being. The goal in Yoga Nidra is to strengthen what isn't 'broken'. When we focus on and strengthen what isn't 'broken', what is 'broken' begins to dissipate and no longer dominates thought forms and lifestyle choices. The practice utilizes an attitude of welcoming. Welcoming presence invites the whole self as whole and begins to integrate one's entire sense of self into feeling whole and complete. This occurs through rewiring neural networks and practices such as pairing positive and negatives with compassion and kindness being to stimulate the network repairs.

Regarding treatment, most treatments begin with showing "what is wrong with me" where yoga nidra and other meditation practices invites us to meet what is not wrong but what is whole. For someone struggling with trauma, depression, anxiety, and physical limitations it is easy to begin to identify with what is wrong, however, yoga nidra begins with what lies beneath those circumstances and heightens our knowing of what is right within us. Over time and practice, this shows up in the participants through less reactivity, self regulation, self care, better communication, and lifestyle choices that are effective to living healthy and well.

In this mindful meditation, when pain arises one is directed to meet the pain with a welcoming presence and compassion. Understanding that we can either use pain to source more pain or see pain as a path to our source, this is how we use the mind to change the mind. Again, pain is inevitable but suffering is optional. Yoga Nidra has been proven to decrease perception of pain, interpersonal discord (feelings of shame, guilt, etc.), PTSD, depression, fear, stress, and insomnia. By planting seeds within the subconscious mind and returning to that intention while in yoga nidra, it becomes possible to recover the nature of who you are at essence and begin to improve outlook and perception based on that inner knowing.

How to practice Yoga Nidra:

Yoga Nidra can either be read to you or you can listen to a recording. I have provided a yoga nidra script to follow along to or for your provider, therapist, loved one, or friend to read to you. You may also record yourself reading it and begin to listen to that recording. There are many yoga nidra recordings online or for sale, and you may even be able to find a yoga nidra class in your local community.

Yoga Nidra encompasses introduction, grounding, intention setting, body scan, breath awareness, sensory awareness,, visualization, and return. Yoga Nidra is a systematic method of complete relaxation and meditation done in a lying position supported by props and blankets used to induce the relaxation response in the body. Make yourself comfortable and enjoy! And if you fall asleep, it happens, so don't worry too much if you fall asleep because the subconscious is always listening.

This script is intended to be read to the patient.

Introduction

To begin Yoga Nidra, you should be lying on your back. Your knees may be slightly bent and supported for comfort within the lower back. Make sure that you are warm enough and that you are in a position that will be comfortable through the duration of the practice. Let your body begin to soften and feel that effortless weight of your body sinking into the floor. Grounded. Feel your breath, letting go of where you came from and where you are going- but grounding into this moment and only this moment. It is best that you remain still during Yoga Nidra so that both your body and mind may fully relax. However, if you become uncomfortable, please change position into one that will be comfortable for this practice. Allow your eyes to close and keep them closed until the practice has ended.

The practice of yoga nidra is a practice of yogic sleep that will guide you to a state of consciousness between wakefulness and sleeping. Imagine that it is a way of coming home to yourself. Try to remain awake by listening to the sound of my voice. If the mind becomes overactive with thoughts and worries, just come back to the sound of my voice. You will be asked to move your awareness to bodily sensations, emotions and images. Try not to concentrate too intensely, simply be aware. During this meditation, please use and absorb what you need in the present moment and leave the rest behind.

Relaxation

Bring your awareness to any sounds you can hear in this moment. Begin to focus on the sounds you hear. Try not to label the source but simply follow each sound, bringing your attention to the most distant sounds you hear. Let your sense of hearing radiate outward, noticing the distant sounds. Then follow each sound to a closer sound from sounds outside this building, to sounds inside this building, to sounds inside this room. Notice the sound of your natural breath flowing in and out of the nose. Now imagine as you gently breathe in infusing the body with vitality, strength, and peace. As you gently exhale out allow anything that may not be serving you in this moment to flush out of the body. Breathing in softly. Breathing out softly. Witnessing your breath.

Feel how the breath oscillates with the movement and flow of your body. Notice the rhythm you feel within your body.

Without opening your eyes visualize the room you are lying in, the ceiling, the floor, and where you are lying. Visualize the position of your body in this moment, your hair, your clothes, your face. Just become aware of your whole body in this moment.

Redirect your awareness back to your breath. The rhythm and flow of your natural breath. The sound almost mimicking the sound of the ocean waves, brushing onto the shore and being pulled back to sea. Maybe notice how it flows from the top of your head down to your feet on the exhale and from the feet to the top of your head on the inhale. Your breath is an expression of your vitality. Gentle breath, slowly into the nose, and even slower out the nose.

Now begin to cultivate your intention for this practice. It should be a short statement in simple language such as I am peaceful, gratitude, self care, surrender, or a wish for yourself from yourself. The intention created in Yoga Nidra plants a seed within the fertile soil of your mind to yield peace and healing through self awareness and surrender. State your intention to yourself clearly and with awareness three times.

Remind yourself, "I am practicing Yoga Nidra, I am relaxed and aware."

Now, we will begin a voyage of sensory awareness throughout your body. You will move your awareness to different parts of your body as soon as you hear them named. Please say the name of the part to yourself and feel that part of your body, but do not move any part. The practice begins on the right side.

Right hand thumb ... 2nd finger ... 3rd finger ... 4th finger ... 5th finger ... palm of the hand ... back of the hand ... wrist ... forearm ... elbow ... upper arm ... shoulder ... armpit ... waist ... hip ... thigh ... knee ... calf ... ankle ... heel ... sole of the foot ... top of the foot ... right big toe ... 2nd toe ... 3rd toe ... 4th toe ... 5th toe.

Left hand thumb ... 2nd finger ... 3rd finger ... 4th finger ... 5th finger ... palm of the hand ... back of the hand ... wrist ... forearm ... elbow ... upper arm ... shoulder ... armpit ... waist ... hip ... thigh ...

knee ... calf ... ankle ... heel ... sole of the foot ... top of the foot ... left big toe ... 2nd toe ... 3rd toe ... 4th toe ... 5th toe.

Now draw your awareness to the back of the body ... right heel ... left heel ... right calf ... left calf ... right thigh ... left thigh ... right buttock ... left buttock ... lower back ... middle back ... upper back ... the entire spine ... right shoulder blade ... left shoulder blade ... back of the neck ... back of the head.

Top of the head ... forehead ... right temple ... left temple ... right ear ... left ear ... right eyebrow ... left eyebrow ... the space between the eyebrows ... right eye ... left eye ... nose ... right cheek ... left cheek ... upper lip ... lower lip ... both lips together ... chin ... jaw ... throat ... right collarbone ... left collar bone ... right side of the chest ... left side of the chest ... upper abdomen ... navel ... lower abdomen ... right groin ... left groin ... the pelvic floor.

The whole right leg ... whole left leg ... whole right arm ... whole left arm ... the whole face ... the whole head ... the whole torso ... pour your awareness into the right side of your body ... pour your awareness into the left side of the body ... feel awareness within the whole body ... the whole body ... the whole body. You are a complete entity of awareness and light.

Opposite Sensations

Lightness/Heaviness:

Now imagine the whole body filled with lightness. As though your body is free, easy, and light. Your body feels as though could float away from the floor and toward the ceiling. Completely light and weightless. The head is light and weightless, the limbs are light and weightless, the heart is light and weightless, the whole body is light and weightless. You are free and weightless.

Now imagine your body becoming heavy. Feel the grounded heaviness in all parts of the body, each part is becoming heavier and heavier and heavier. The head is heavy, the limbs are heavy, the whole body is heavy. So heavy that you feel your body grounding down into the floor. You are so heavy, grounding deeper and deeper.

Cold/Hot:

Now begin to stir the experience of cold within the body, the experience of icy cold permeating your entire body. As though you feel an achy wind chilling you to your bones.

Now allow the sensation of warmth to spread throughout the entire body. Comforting warmth radiating from the bones to your skin as if the sun is beating down upon you illuminating you with its rays. You feel a glowing warmth all around the body.

Witnessing Space Visualization

Begin to notice the blank space in front of your closed eyelids. Notice any sensations, patterns, colors, or light within this mind screen but do not become involved in directing, controlling, or identifying what you see. This is the manifesting state of your consciousness so invite yourself to become a witness of your experience. Become a witness of your awareness. Practicing this with detached awareness only.

Now we are going to navigate through visualizations allowing each to arise on your mental screen. Notice each visualization; whether through imagery, feeling, smell, or sound of each experience.

Burning candle ... Burning candle ... Burning candle ... peacock feather ... peacock feather ... peacock feather ... tall tree... tall tree ... tall tree ... swing on a porch ... swing on a porch ... swing on a porch ... heavy rain ... heavy rain ... heavy rain ... a beautiful garden path ... a beautiful garden path ... and beautiful garden path ... moving clouds ... moving clouds ... moving clouds ... starlit night ... starlit night ... starlit night ... full moon ... full moon ... full moon ... sleeping cat ... sleeping cat ... sleeping cat ... fish swimming ... fish swimming ... fish swimming ... galloping horse ... galloping horse ... galloping horse ... vibrant sunset ... vibrant sunset ... vibrant sunset ... river flowing ... river flowing ... river flowing ... foggy morning ... foggy morning ... foggy morning ... waterfall in a mountain ... waterfall in a mountain ... waterfall in a mountain ... a field of flowers ... a field of flowers ...

a field of flowers ... yourself in deep meditation ... yourself in deep meditation ... yourself in deep meditation

Return

It is time to repeat your intention. Please repeat the same statement made at the beginning of the practice three times mentally now.

Come back to the feeling of your breath flowing in and out of your nostrils. The feeling of your breath flowing in and out of your body. Your body is relaxed and comfortable. Feel the container of your skin and the sensations that which are touching you. Notice the heaviness of your body as it rests on the floor and take your awareness into all the points that are touching the floor. Without opening your eyes, direct your awareness to your whole body and to your surroundings. Taking your time, begin to wiggle the toes and fingers. When you feel yourself begin to fully awake gently open your eyes and bring your knees into your chest rocking side to side. Please roll over to whatever side is comfortable to you. Stay on your side for a few more moments taking a deep breath in and sigh it out. Use your hands to press yourself up from the floor and let your head come up last.

The practice of Yoga Nidra is now complete.

CONCLUSION

Welcome Yourself Home

~~~~~~~

"And remember, no matter where you go, there you are." -Confucius

The intention of this book has been to delineate and apply the chakra modality in conjunction with everyday living and health intervention. To generate "aha!" moments and to realize that there is not a light at the end of the tunnel, because you control the light- let this serve as a reminder to turn it on. The more we keep searching for relief and peace outside of ourselves, the more we are left feeling lonely, exhausted, and unfulfilled thus leading to illness. Suffering, however, is the catalyst to transformation. Through connecting yourself to the chakra story, the imbalances, and solutions; you have begun to find direction and confidence in moving through your own labyrinth of healing. Confidence is a by product of clarity - to know and act in courage. It is about tapping into our own entelechy to flourish into the best and most healed versions of ourselves, to create a healthy life, and to liberate ourselves from avoidable suffering.

The chakra continuum expounds the process of creation and liberation. We are first inspired (7th chakra) into contemplation. We think on that inspiration and then hold vision for it(6th chakra). Then it moves into speaking to actualize (5th chakra) the inspiration thus moving into devotion (4th chakra) and serving that inspiration. By devotion comes power (3rd chakra) to vitalize the inspiration. Through power, it becomes creatively (2nd chakra) alchemized into a manifested state (1st chakra). Creatives, innovators, teachers, physicians, and people of all walks use this creation blueprint when solving problems or creating an impact; all energetically flowing from the chakras. By understanding this process we can utilize it more consciously and effectively to empower our choices.

There is no easy quick fix to anything that remains sustainable. One cannot simply bask in a purple bath or hold designated crystals or even depend on medications alone. The most sustainable healing practice is cultivated through lifestyle choices, eating habits, environment, movement, sociality, and mental thought form. Living holistically involves intentional thoughts and deliberate action, therefore, creating an optimal experience each day, moment by moment, breath by breath.

The ultimate health continuum should embody promotion, prevention, treatment, recovery, and maintenance. It begins with promotion and education in order to equip the individual and public with self-sustainable tools and knowledge that encourage individuals to make sustainable choices that enable a healthier life. This leads to strengthening health prevention initiatives that would decrease healthcare costs where allopathic medicine no longer becomes known as disease management, but serves the role it was intended as. Treatment would exist as a way to actually treat patients supporting their rehabilitation and would recuperate the individual back into optimal health and wellness prepared for maintenance beyond recovery.

At the end of the day, everything comes down to choice. Each choice made, holds accountability and responsibility for the experiences and entities impacted. It is easy to neglect our bodies, especially when we become overwhelmed with the flow of daily tasks. As we begin to understand that the capacity of our living is in relationship to our mind and body, we create the grounds to make supportive choices. When our whole being is off-balance, fatigued, and neglected, we begin to manifest disease that can spread as a repercussion in other areas of our life. Whatever initiative taken to promote self-healing and a balanced life comes down to our decisions and actions. Our body was created to support us and holds an innate design for living. The more you learn about your body's physical, mental, and spiritual nature, the more you can react in ways to prevent illness and rise through ailments- both utilizing the holistic platform of intuition and choice. Offer yourself compassion when needed but also offer yourself accountability when appropriate. We are really the only ones who can know the experience of living in our own flesh; thus, we have the power to make it vibrantly sustainable. Though we each possess an innate design for understanding, healing, and abundance - providence is simply the canvas, you create the art.

YOGA POSE GLOSSARY

First Chakra:

Garland Pose- (squat)

Stand with feet a little further than hip distance and begin to forward fold bending the knees and dropping the pelvis towards the ground. Sink into the hips slowly. Meet yourself where it feels comfortable. If this is too much for your hips, maybe find Chair pose and breathe there. Your heels may or may not touch the ground. It makes no difference, again meet yourself where you are.

Bridge (focus into the gluts, pelvic floor)-

Lying on your back with your knees in your chest, begin to let your feet come down to the mat walking your feet closer to the glutes. Press into the feet lifting the pelvis up strengthening through your low back and glutes. This pose is also wonderful for low back pain. As you are here, begin to breathe in and out of the nose slowly focusing on your pelvis region and pelvic floor. Hold for thirty seconds to one minute. Once you are finished slowly lower each vertebrae down at a time until your whole spine is on the ground. Pull your knees into your chest, giving yourself a hug and rock side to side.

Forward Fold-

With your feet a little wider than hip width apart, begin to take your hands down the front of your legs finding a forward fold. Let your arms relax, or cross your arms holding onto your elbows. Let the head completely hang, the spine completely hang. Being to shift your weight into the right and left foot gently swaying side to side, or be still. Make this yours. Feel gravity pulling and opening the spine as your relax the face and the jaw. Surrender here, let the eyes close or soften.

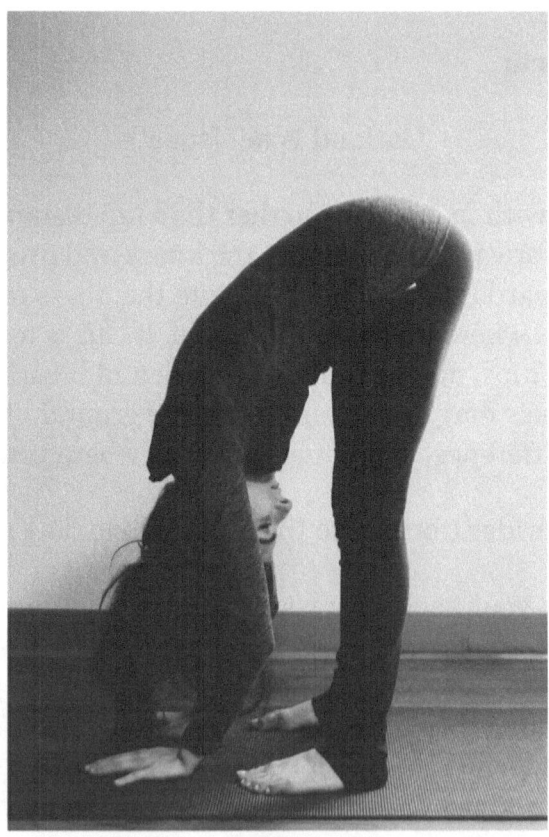

Second Chakra

Child's Pose

Come onto your hands and knees and sink your hips back allowing your body to soften over your thigh. You can either take your knees wide or keep them together but feel the weight of your hips and tailbone lengthening the spine as you rest over your knees. You can take a pillow between your knees if it helps your torso feel more supported. Relax your arms either in front of you or at your sides. If you would like begin to move your hips side to side or making fluid like movements with your hips.

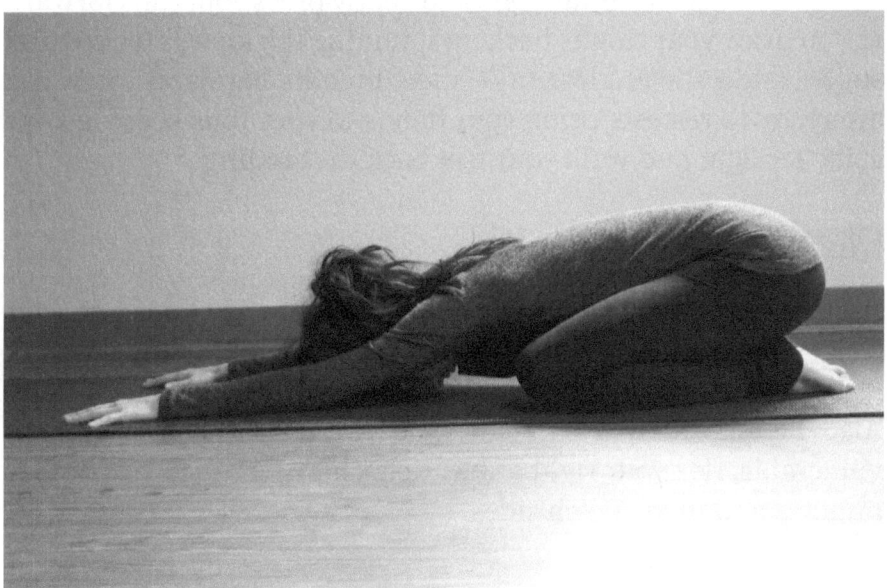

Restorative: Legs up the wall

Sit with your side against the wall. Roll back sliding your side against the wall and then swivel your body so your legs roll up onto the wall as you lie on your back. Relax here. This pose is also known to help with low back pain, migraines, anxiety, varicose veins, and circulation.

Goddess Pose

Begin in a standing position with your arms at your side. Bring your hands to rest comfortably on your hips. Begin to step your feet apart so you are standing with wide legs. Turn your toes out slightly so they point at an angle. Take a breath in through the nose and on the exhale begin to bend your knees so the knees are stacked above the ankles. Work towards bringing your thighs parallel to the floor, but honor your body and do not force yourself into a squat. Extend your arms out with your palms facing down and then rotate your palms facing up. Bend your elbows at a 90 degree angle with palms face up towards the sky softening the shoulders.. Tuck your tailbone and gently press your hips forward as you draw your thighs back maintaining the knees stacked and stable above the ankles. Take a few breaths here and when you are ready to release, bring your hands to your hips keeping your spine straight and walk your feet back to standing.

Pigeon Pose

Begin in downward facing dog and draw your right knee into your chest lowering it down and sinking into the hips feeling your left leg slide back. If this is uncomfortable try reclined pigeon pose. Also, be mindful of your right knee. If it feels uncomfortable or vulnerable, flex your right ankle. Relax here for about two or four minutes and then switch sides.

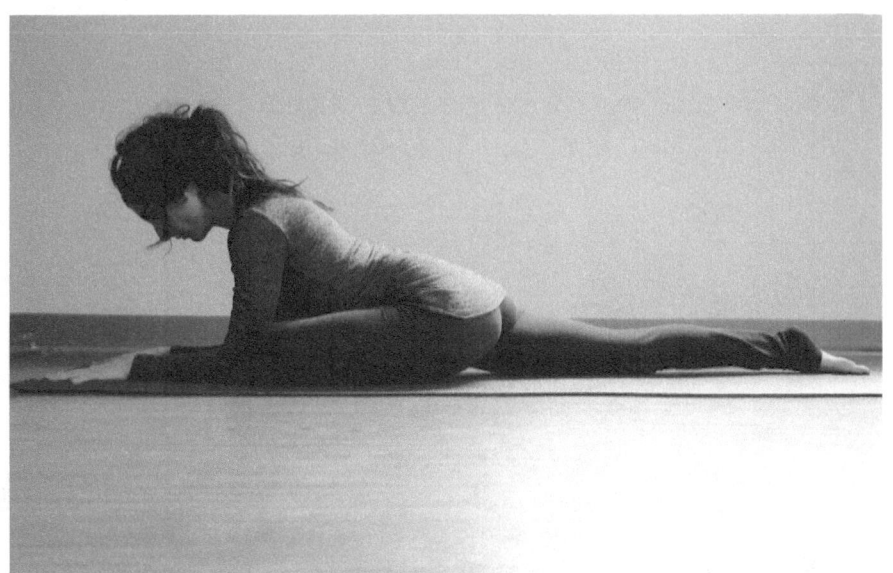

Reclined Pigeon Pose

Lay on your back with both knees in your chest. Slightly lengthen your right leg and bend your left knee drawing it in. Bring the right leg up and take your left hand between your legs, the right hand around the right leg and interlace fingers pulling the right leg in. If you need a strap to connect your hands use that.

If both of those hip stretches are uncomfortable try this seated. Coming to the edge of a chair with your feet planted on the ground. Begin to take the right leg, bend the right knee, and cross your shin over the top of the left knee (so it rests on the left thigh above the left knee) while the left foot is still planted on the ground. If your right leg cannot cross over the left leg, lengthen the left leg out to cross. Ideally, you would want the outside of the right ankle to rest on the top of the left thigh. Once you are here, notice if you feel a hip stretch. If it is subtle and you would like more of a stretch, begin to lean forward until you find a stretch comfortable to you. Hold for one minute. Switch sides.

Bound Angle

In a comfortable seat, bring the soles of your feet together and slowly lean forward keeping your spine lengthened.

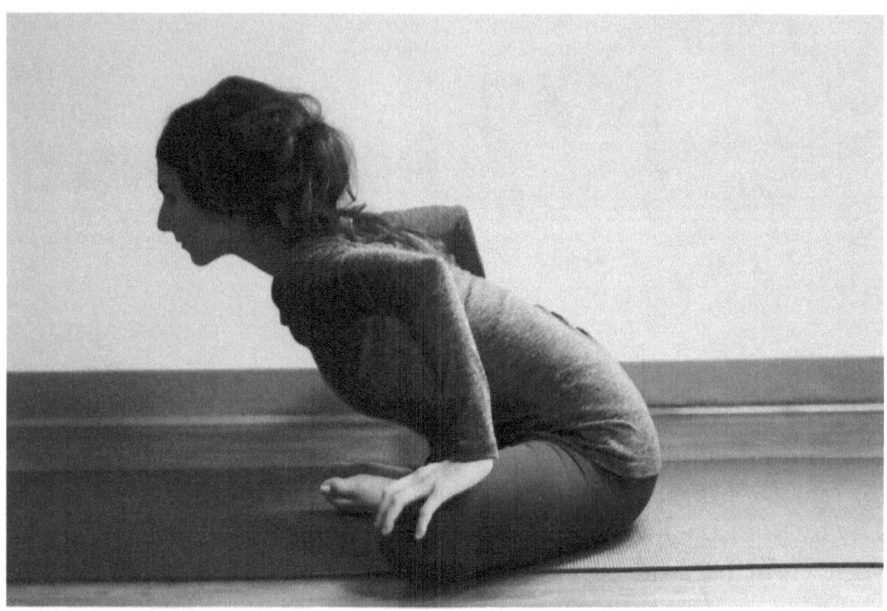

Tabletop fluid movements-

Coming onto your hands and knees, begin to draw circles with your hips moving freely here. Utilizing intuitive movement pivoting from the knees and the wrists. It is almost like using your bones to massage the body from the inside out. You may move freely into anything direction or movement that feels good for you.

Third Chakra:

Spinal Rotations

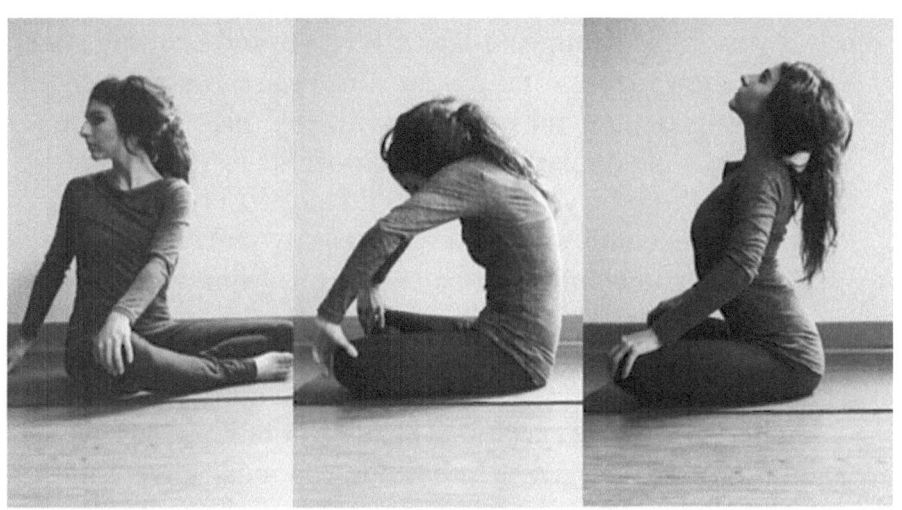

twist, forward fold, backbend

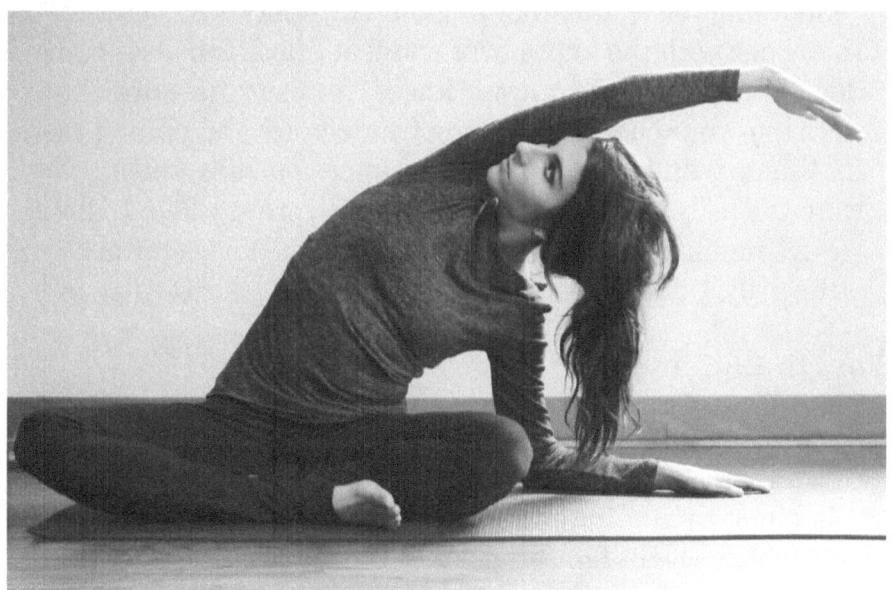

Side bends

Boat Pose

Begin seated on the floor with your legs lengthened in front of you. Take a breath in and then on the exhale slowly lean back at your hips lifting your legs off the ground bending your knees just a few inches off the floor. Once you feel stable, begin to slowly straighten out your legs with your arms reaching out in front of you parallel to the floor. Engage your core here. From the side, your body should look like a V. Hold for ten to thirty seconds and then when you're ready bring your legs down, come onto your back, and give yourself a hug.

Sun Salutations

There are many variations of sun salutations. Sun salutations are energizing and generate a meditative, fluid movement where the body can flow through the poses while the mind and body are linked yoked together.

Soothing the Abdominal Region with Viniyoga Exercise: Lie on back with the knees bent and feet lifted. Inhale and arms lengthen with hands on your knees. On the exhale draw the knees into your chest by bending your elbows and pulling them in. Inhale with hands still on your knees pushing knees away from the belly so the knees and low back are stacked. Exhale, with hands still on the knees drawing the knees towards the belly. Continue this meditative flow at your own pace.

Fourth Chakra:

Triangle Pose

Begin in a standing wide legged pose. Starting with the right side, pivot the right foot 90 degrees so it is perpendicular to the left. Begin to slowly take the right hand and drop it down below the knee, ideally towards the right ankle. Draw in the core as you lengthen the spine and extend the left arm up to the sky pulling the shoulder back so the heart begins to open. You can either let your head face down towards the right foot or gaze up at the left hand, whichever is more comfortable for your neck. Feel the side body stretch engaging the core to stabilize the pelvis. Do not let your right hand rest on the right knee. Also, do not allow your body weight to drop into the right arm. Be mindful of over extending the right arm, so use the core to hold your body weight. Breathe here for a few breaths and then switch sides.

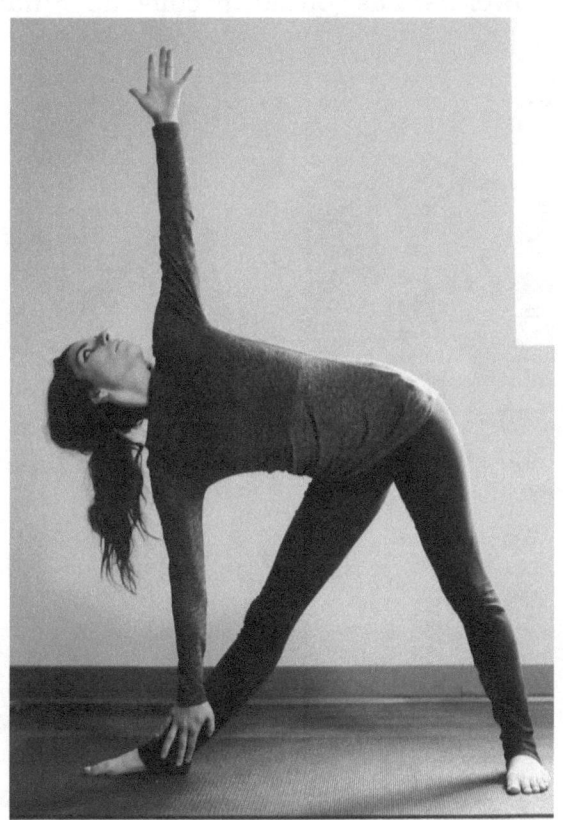

Camel

Come onto your knees and take your hands to your low back. Begin to press your hips forward as you gentle begin to sink back into a backbend. One variation is simply keeping your hands pressed into your low back as you get a back bend gentle letting the head drop back. The second is once you've begun to drop into your back bend, take your right hand to the right ankle and the left hand to the left ankle. Once you are here send the hips forward keeping the core engaged and the chest raised peeling the shoulders back. Let the head and neck relax back. Be mindful of your breath and if this pose is uncomfortable, come out of it immediately. To come out of the pose, bring your chin back towards your chest and your hands to your low back. Engage the lower belly and your hands to support your lower back as you slowly come up. Find child's pose and rest.

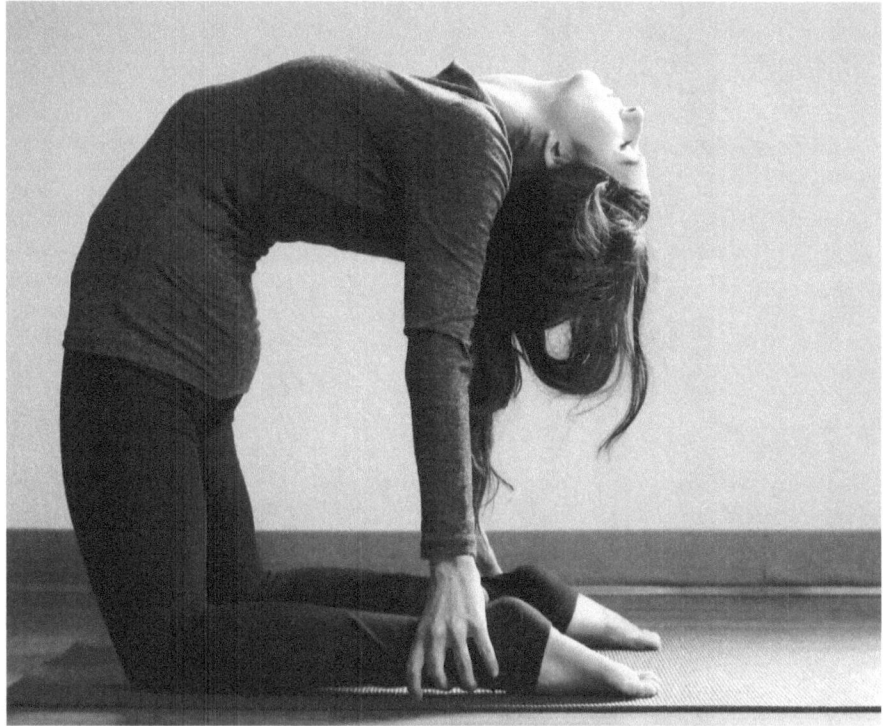

Supported Reclined Bound Angle

With the soles of your feet together, begin to recline back onto a blanket or bolster along your spine allowing your body to relax here. Close the eyes and breathing in and out through the nose feeling the breath climb the spine and gently relax opening the chest further and further with each exhale.

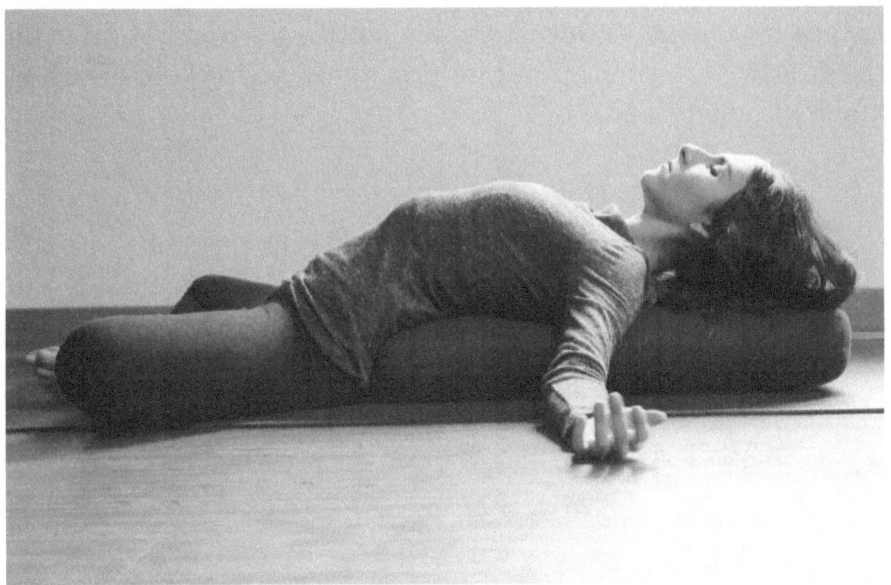

Heart Opening Flow

You can do this either seated or standing. Begin to bend your elbows and pull the shoulders back, down, and back finding cactus arms. Take a deep breath in and as you exhale draw your elbows or hands together. Inhale, opening back into cactus arms. Exhale, rounding the spine drawing the elbows or hands together. Continue this with your breath.

Fifth Chakra:

Bridge Pose

Lying on your back with your knees bent and feet planted on the ground. Begin to walk your feet closer to the glutes to stabilize the low back. Press into the feet lifting the pelvis up strengthening through your low back and glutes. Allow your arms to stay relaxed by your side, strengthening through the glutes to support the body. Notice the throat region. As you are here, begin to breathe in and out of the nose slowly focusing on the sensations within the throat. Hold for one minute. Once you are finished slowly lower each vertebrae down at a time until your whole spine is on the ground. Pull your knees into your chest, giving yourself a hug and rock side to side.

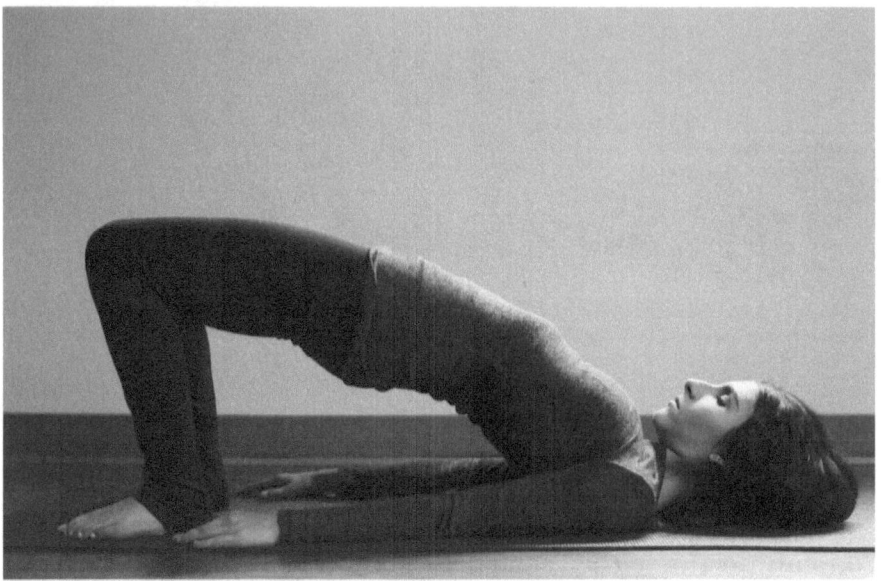

Shoulder Stand

Shoulder stand is an inversion that stimulates the thyroid gland and opens the shoulders and neck. If you have limitations within the neck, fold one or two towels under your body so that your head rests just off the edge of the folded towel onto the floor with your shoulders and arms on the towel. If this pose doesn't feel right, refrain from doing it.

Begin by lying on your back with your knees bent, feet flat on the floor. Take a breath in and then on the exhale, bend your knees and draw your thighs up towards the belly. Engage the core muscles as you lift your bottom off the floor and place your hands on your low back to begin to straighten the legs towards the sky. Stabilize yourself by drawing in your core and extending through the toes. Allow the face, neck, and shoulders to soften. Notice your breath. Your elbows should be planted onto the floor with your hands pressed into the flow back. Stay here as long as you'd like. When you are ready to come down slowly begin to draw your knees in using your hands to slowly lower you down, coming down each vertebrae at a time. Hug your knees into your chest and breathe.

Plow Pose

Be mindful of where you are. If this pose doesn't feel right to you, be patient and begin with practicing spinal flexibility. During this position you may need to use a folded towel to place beneath your shoulders for better support.

Begin by lying on your back with your arms by your side. Take a breath in and then on the exhale, bend your knees and draw your thighs up towards the belly. Engage the core muscles as you lift your bottom off the floor and place your hands on your low back to begin to straighten the legs upward. Stabilize yourself and allow the face, neck, and shoulders to soften. Notice your breath. Once you have softened and feel stable begin to drop one leg behind your head and if you feel comfortable drop the other leg behind your head. Hold this posture for a few breaths and feel the energy within the throat chakra.

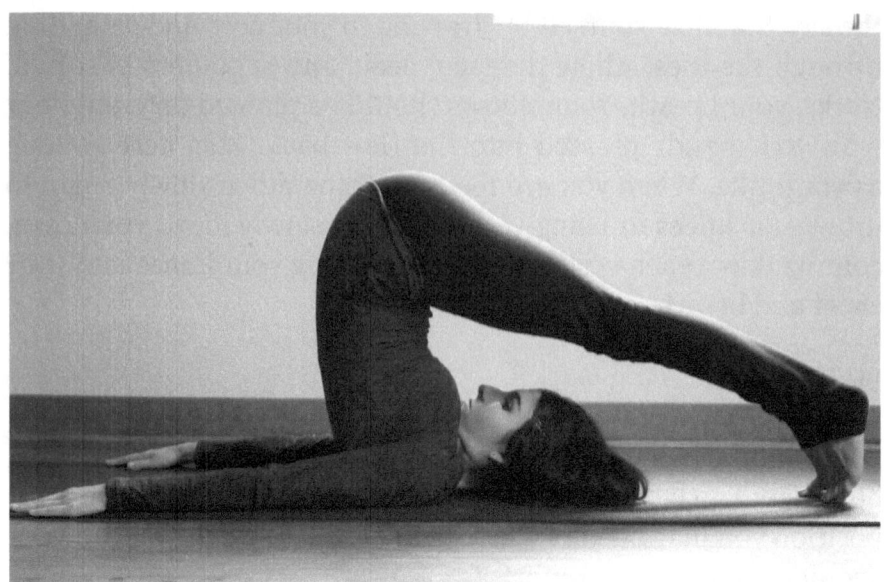

Neck Rolls

Begin in a comfortable position. Take a breath in throat the nose and then exhale the chin towards the chest. Inhale the right ear towards the right shoulder, then exhale chin to chest. Inhale the left ear towards the left shoulder, then exhale chin to chest. Repeat this while paying attention to the sensation and stretch within the neck. Allow the breath to initiate the movement and if you begin to crave free movement within the neck- tune in and move freely opening the muscles of the neck. If you feel tension, maybe pause there and breath into it. Practice for one minute.

Sixth Chakra:

Child's pose with forehead to the floor.

Rocking the head gently side to side also stimulates a nice massage onto the forehead.

Downward Facing Dog

Come onto your hands and knees, begin to tuck the toes lifting the hips to the sky. Notice your hands pressed into the mat and begin to push into your hands as though you are pushing the mat out from beneath you. Let the head relax.

Down Dog helps increase blood flow into the head. Relax the neck and breath using this pose to calm the mind and energize the whole body.

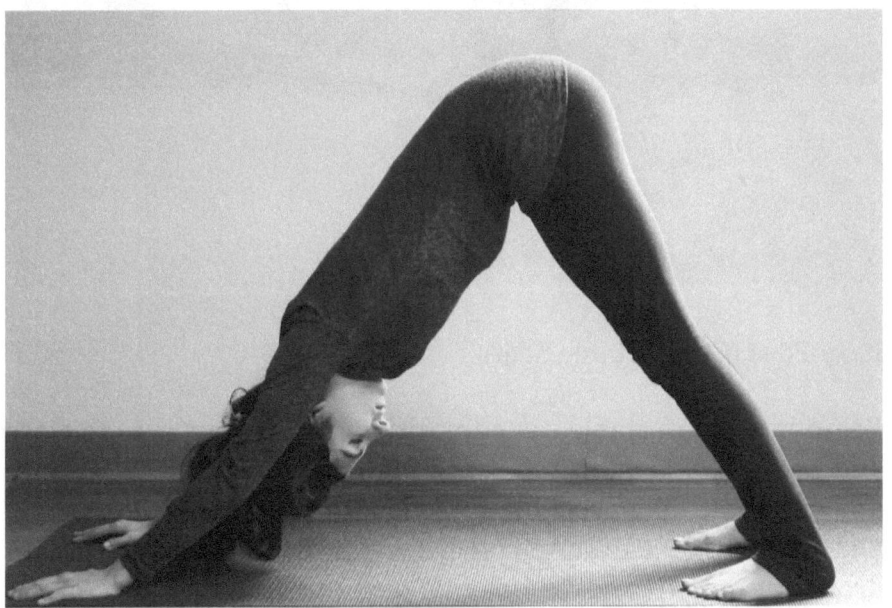

Seventh Chakra:

Savasana or Relaxation pose

This pose is the posed used at the end of a yoga practice to relax the body and absorb all the benefits of the practice. It is the most important poses in the yoga practice because it allows you to absorb the practice and its benefits. Relaxation pose helps lower blood pressure, reduces headache, fatigue, stress, and insomnia.

The ideal time frame of savasana is between seven to twenty minutes. Make yourself cozy and drop into your body, surrender.

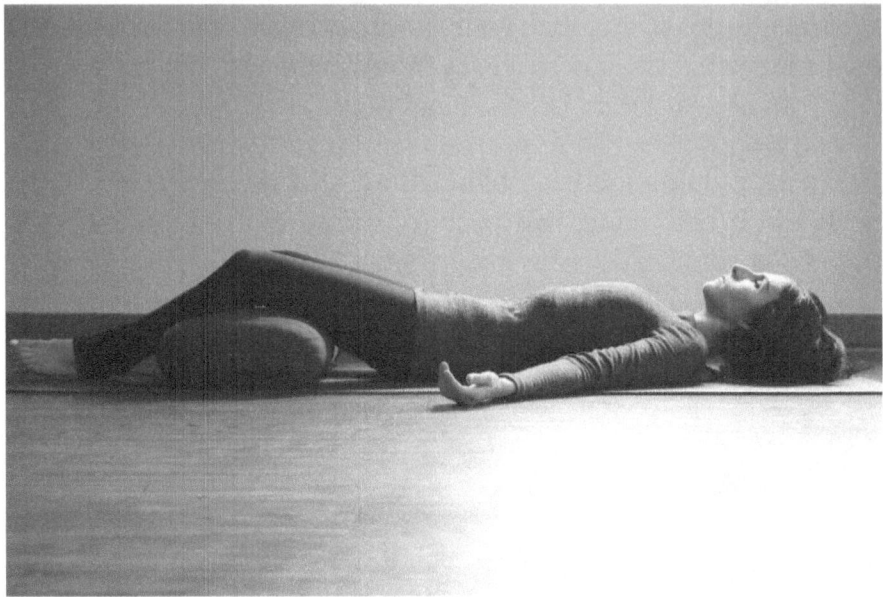

Easy Pose (Comfortable Seat)

Begin in a comfortable seated position. Allow your eyes to close and begin to focus on the sensation of your breath flowing in and out of the body. Feel the spine lengthen up with every inhale and allow the face to soften on every exhale. Notice as the breath draws in warmth, maybe imagine being filled with light. As you attend this moment, notice the expansiveness of the body lifting taller towards the sky. Feel whole here, feel alive. Practice this for at least one minute.

INDEX

Preface

Gerteis J, Izrael D, Deitz D, LeRoy L, Ricciardi R, Miller T, Basu J. Multiple Chronic Conditions Chartbook.[PDF - 10.62 MB] AHRQ Publications No, Q14-0038. Rockville, MD: Agency for Healthcare Research and Quality; 2014. Accessed November 18, 2014.

Keshet, Y. "Dual Embedded Agency: Physicians Implement Integrative Medicine in Health-care Organizations." *Health: An Interdisciplinary Journal for the Social Study of Health, Illness and Medicine* 17.6 (2013): 605-21. Web.

Lasater JH. Down the road: yoga therapy in the future. Int J Yoga Ther. 2010.

McCall, Timothy B. *Yoga as Medicine: The Yogic Prescription for Health & Healing: A Yoga Journal Book.* New York: Bantam, 2007. Print.

"Waste in the Health Care System." *The New York Times*. The New York Times, 10 Sept. 2012. Web. 15 Sept. 2015.

Chronic Illness

Bock, Beth C., et al. "Yoga as a complementary treatment for smoking cessation in women." *Journal of Women's Health* 21.2 (2012): 240-248.

Centers for Disease Control and Prevention. Exercise or Physical Activity. NCHS FastStats Web site. http://www.cdc.gov/nchs/fastats/exercise.htm. Accessed December 20, 2013.

Hyman, Mark A., Dean Ornish, and Michael Roizen. "Lifestyle medicine: treating the causes of disease." *Alternative Therapies in Health & Medicine* 15.6 (2009): 12.

McIver, Shane, Paul O'Halloran, and Michael McGartland. "The impact of Hatha yoga on smoking behavior." *Alternative therapies in health and medicine* 10.2 (2004): 22.

Ornish, Dean. *Dr. Dean Ornish's program for reversing heart disease*. Ivy books, 2010.

Ornish, Dean, Gerdi Weidner, William R. Fair, Ruth Marlin, Elaine B. Pettengill, Caren J. Raisin, Stacey Dunn-Emke, Lila Crutchfield, F. Nicholas Jacobs, and R. James Barnard. "Intensive Lifestyle Changes May Affect The Progression Of Prostate Cancer." *The Journal of Urology* 174.3 (2005): 1065-070. Web.

Pope, Sandra K., Valorie M. Shue, and Cornelia Beck. "Will a healthy lifestyle help prevent Alzheimer's disease?." *Annual Review of Public Health* 24.1 (2003): 111-132.

Schwartz, Jerome L. "Smoking cures: Ways to kick an unhealthy habit." *Research on smoking behavior* (1977): 308.

"Yoga May Guard against Heart Disease, Study Finds - BBC News." *BBC News*. N.p., n.d. Web. 10 Nov. 2015.

Holism

Strandberg EL, Ovhed I, Borgquist L, et al; The perceived meaning of a (w)holistic view among general practitioners and BMC Fam Pract. 2007 Mar 8;8:8.

Kabat-Zinn, Jon. Introduction. *Full Catastrophe Living: Using the Wisdom of Your Body and Mind to Face Stress, Pain, and Illness*. New York, NY: Pub. by Dell Pub., a Division of Bantam Doubleday Dell Pub. Group, 1991. 12. Print.

Medical Lens

Fadlon, J. "Meridians, Chakras and Psycho-Neuro-Immunology: The Dematerializing Body and the Domestication of Alternative Medicine." *Body & Society* 10.4 (2004): 69-86. Web.

Maxwell, R. W. (2009), THE PHYSIOLOGICAL FOUNDATION OF YOGA CHAKRA EXPRESSION. Zygon, 44: 807–824. doi: 10.1111/j.1467-9744.2009.01035.x

1

Bock, Beth C., Joseph L. Fava, Ronnesia Gaskins, Kathleen M. Morrow, David M. Williams, Ernestine Jennings, Bruce M. Becker, Geoffrey Tremont, and Bess H. Marcus. "Yoga as a Complementary Treatment for Smoking Cessation in Women." *Journal of Women's Health* 21.2 (2012): 240-48. Web.

Gelderloos P, Walton KG, Orme-Johnson DW, Alexander CN. Effectiveness of Transcendental Meditation program in preventing and treating substance misuse; a review. Int J Addict 1991

Iyengar, B. K. S. *Light on Yoga: Yoga Dipika.* New York: Schocken, 1979. Print.

Littlejohn, Darren. *The 12-step Buddhist: Enhance Recovery from Any Addiction.* Hillsboro, Or.: Beyond Words Pub., 2009. Print.

Raina N, Chakraborty PK, Basit MA, et al. Evaluation of yoga therapy in alcohol dependence. Indian Journal of Psychiatry. 2001

"RenewEveryday.com." *Addiction & Recovery Statistics.* N.p., n.d. Web. 10 Nov. 2015.

Services, Inc Alcoholics Anonymous World. *Alcoholics Anonymous: The Big Book --4th Ed.--.* New York City, NY: Alcoholics Anonymous World Services, 2001. Print.

Trivette, Evan T., Kyle Hoedebecke, Cristóbal S. Berry-Cabán, and Brandy R. Jacobs. "Megaloblastic Hematopoiesis in a 20 Year Old Pregnant Female." *The American Journal of Case Reports.* International Scientific Literature, Inc., n.d. Web. 10 Nov. 2015.

"Yoga as a Complementary Treatment for Smoking Cessation in Women." *National Center for Biotechnology Information.* U.S. National Library of Medicine, n.d. Web. <http://www.ncbi.nlm.nih.gov/pubmed/21992583>.

2nd Chakra

"ARMY.MIL, The Official Homepage of the United States Army." *Traumatic Brain Injury Awareness Month Highlights Resources.* N.p., 12 Feb. 2015. Web. <http://www.army.mil/article/142825>.

Batten SV, Orsillo SM, Walser RD. Acceptance and mindfulness-based approaches to the treatment of posttraumatic stress disorder. In: Orsillo SM, Roemer L, eds *Acceptance and Mindfulness-Based Approaches to Anxiety.* New York, NY: Springer US; 2005.

Bedard M, Felteau M, Mazmanian D, et al. Pilot evaluation of a mindfulness-based intervention to improve quality of life among individuals who sustained traumatic brain injuries. Disabil Rehab. 2003.

Berceli, David. *The Revolutionary Trauma Release Process: Transcend Your Toughest times.* Vancouver: Namaste Pub., 2008. Print.

Briere, John, and Catherine Scott. *Principles of Trauma Therapy: A Guide to Symptoms, Evaluation, and Treatment.* Los Angeles: Sage Publications, 2013. Print.

Cappo BM, Holmes DS. The utility of prolonged respiratory exhalation for reducing physiological and psychological arousal in non-threatening and threatening situations. J Psychosomatic Res. 1984.

Disorder: A Randomized Controlled Pilot Study." *Journal of Clinical Psychology J. Clin. Psychol.*69.1 (2012): 14-27. Web.

"Effectiveness of a Meditation-based Stress Reduction Program in the Treatment of Anxiety Disorders." *American Journal of Psychiatry AJP*149.7 (1992): 936-43. Web.

Groessl EJ, Weingart KR, Aschbacher K, Pada L, Baxi S. Yoga for veterans with chronic low-back pain. J Altern Complement Med 2008.

Frayne S, Chiu V, Iqbal S, et al. Medical care needs of returning veterans with PTSD; their other burden. J Gen Intern Med. 2011.

Herman, Judith Lewis. *Trauma and Recovery.* New York: Basic, 1997. Print.

Jella SA. Shannahoff-Khalsa DS, Kennedy B. The effects of unilateral forced nostril breathing on cognitive performance. Int J Neurosci 1993.

Kearney, David J., Kelly Mcdermott, Carol Malte, Michelle Martinez, and Tracy L. Simpson. "Association of Participation in a Mindfulness Program with Measures of PTSD, Depression and Quality of Life in a Veteran Sample." *Journal of Clinical Psychology J. Clin. Psychol.* 68.1 (2011): 101-16. Web.

Kearney, David J., Kelly Mcdermott, Carol Malte, Michelle Martinez, and Tracy L. Simpson. "Effects of Participation in a Mindfulness Program for Veterans With Posttraumatic Stress

Kolk, Bessel Van Der. "Somatic Therapies for Traumatic Stress." *PsycEXTRA Dataset* (2008): n. pag. Web.

Kolk, Bessel Van Der. "When Talk Isn't Enough." *PsycEXTRA Dataset* (2014): n. pag. Web.

Johansson, B., H. Bjuhr, and L. Rönnbäck. "Mindfulness-based Stress Reduction (MBSR) Improves Long-term Mental Fatigue after Stroke or Traumatic Brain Injury." *Brain Inj Brain Injury* 26.13-14 (2012): 1621-628. Web.

Lee, H. "Yoga Improves Perceived Stress and Psychological Outcomes in Distressed Women." *Focus on Alternative and Complementary Therapies* 18.4 (2013): 217-18. Web.

Libby DJ, Pilver CE, Desai R. Complemntary and alternative medicine use among individuals with PTSD. Pyshcol Trauma: Theory, Res, Pract, Policy. In Press.

Naveen KV, Nagarathna R, Nagendra HR, Telles S. Yoga breathing through a particular nostril increases spatial memory scores without lateralized effects. Psychol Rep. 1997.

Robertson, Kayela, and Maureen Schmitter-Edgecombe. "Self-awareness and Traumatic Brain Injury Outcome." *Brain Injury* 29.7-8 (2015): 848-58. Web.

Shay, Jonathan. *Odysseus in America: Combat Trauma and the Trials of Homecoming*. New York: Scribner, 2002. Print.

Stoller, C. C., J. H. Greuel, L. S. Cimini, M. S. Fowler, and J. A. Koomar. "Effects of Sensory-Enhanced Yoga on Symptoms of Combat Stress in Deployed Military Personnel." *American Journal of Occupational Therapy* 66.1 (2011): 59-68. Web.

Telles, Shirley, Nilkamal Singh, Meesha Joshi, and Acharya Balkrishna. "Post Traumatic Stress Symptoms and Heart Rate Variability in Bihar Flood Survivors following Yoga: A Randomized Controlled Study." *BMC Psychiatry* 10.1 (2010): 18. Web.

"The Veterans Health Administration's Treatment of PTSD and Traumatic Brain Injury Among Recent Combat Veterans." *Congressional Budget Office*. N.p., 09 Feb. 2012. Web. <https://www.cbo.gov/publication/42969>.

3th Chakra

Effectiveness of Shavasana on depression among university students.

Khumar, S. S.; Kaur, Paramjit; Kaur, Sarabjit

Indian Journal of Clinical Psychology, Vol 20(2), Sep 1993, 82-87.

Gershon, Michael D. *The Second Brain: The Scientific Basis of Gut Instinct and a Groundbreaking New Understanding of Nervous Disorders of the Stomach and Intestine*. New York, NY: HarperCollinsPublishers, 1998. Print.

Keefer, L., and E.b Blanchard. "A One Year Follow-up of Relaxation Response Meditation as a Treatment for Irritable Bowel Syndrome." *Behaviour Research and Therapy* 40.5 (2002): 541-46. Web.

Keefer, Laurie, and Edward B. Blanchard. "The Effects of Relaxation Response Meditation on the Symptoms of Irritable Bowel Syndrome: Results of a Controlled Treatment Study." *Behaviour Research and Therapy* 39.7 (2001): 801-11. Web.

Liebler, Nancy Cullen, and Sandra Moss. *Healing Depression the Mind-body Way: Creating Happiness through Meditation, Yoga, and Ayurveda*. Hoboken, NJ: John Wiley, 2009. Print.

Oretzky, Shira, Melanie A. Greenberg, and Richard Baker. "Application of Yoga to Treat Elevated Depressive Symptoms." *PsycEXTRA Dataset*(2007): n. pag. Web.

"Result Filters." *National Center for Biotechnology Information*. U.S. National Library of Medicine, n.d. Web. 10 Nov. 2015.

Weintraub, Amy. *Yoga for Depression: A Compassionate Guide to Relieve Suffering through Yoga*. New York: Broadway, 2004. Print.

Zernicke, Kristin A., Tavis S. Campbell, Philip K. Blustein, Tak S. Fung, Jillian A. Johnson, Simon L. Bacon, and Linda E. Carlson. "Mindfulness-Based Stress Reduction for the Treatment of Irritable Bowel Syndrome Symptoms: A Randomized Wait-list Controlled Trial." *Int.J. Behav. Med. International Journal of Behavioral Medicine* 20.3 (2012): 385-96. Web.

4th Chakra

Adams CE, Leary MR. Promoting self-compassionate attitudes toward eating among restrictive and guilty eaters. Journal of Social and Clinical Psychology. 2007

Boehm, Katja, Thomas Ostermann, Stefania Milazzo, and Arndt Büssing. "Effects of Yoga Interventions on Fatigue: A Meta-Analysis." *Evidence-Based Complementary and Alternative Medicine* 2012 (2012): 1-9. Web.

Cohen, Debbie, and Raymond R. Townsend. "Yoga and Hypertension." *The Journal of Clinical Hypertension* 9.10 (2007): 800-01. Web.

Cohen, Debbie L. "Yoga and Hypertension." *Journal of Yoga & Physical Therapy J Yoga Phys Ther* 03.04 (2013): n. pag. Web.

Dittmann, K. A., and M. R. Freedman. "Body Awareness, Eating Attitudes, and Spiritual Beliefs of Women Practicing Yoga." *Eating Disorders* 17.4 (2009): 273-92. Web.

Farhi, Donna. *The Breathing Book: Good Health and Vitality through Essential Breath Work*. New York: Henry Holt, 1996. Print.

Kiecolt-Glaser, Janice K., Lynanne Mcguire, Theodore F. Robles, and Ronald Glaser. "Psychoneuroimmunology: Psychological Influences on Immune Function and Health." *Journal of Consulting and Clinical Psychology* 70.3 (2002): 537-47. Web.

Leary MR, Tate EB, Adams CE, Allen AB, Hancock J. Self-compassion and reactions to unpleasant self-relavant events: the implications of treating oneself kindly. J Pers Soc Psychol. 2007

http://www.ncbi.nlm.nih.gov/pubmed/17484611

Masin, Pam. "4 Amazing Health Benefits Of Helping Others." *The Huffington Post*. TheHuffingtonPost.com, 28 Dec. 2013. Web. <http://www.huffingtonpost.com/2013/12/28/health-benefits-of-helping-others_n_4427697.html>.

Mizuno, Julio, and Henrique Luiz Monteiro. "An Assessment of a Sequence of Yoga Exercises to Patients with Arterial Hypertension." *Journal of Bodywork and Movement Therapies* 17.1 (2013): 35-41. Web.

Murthy, S.n., N.s.n. Rao, Babina Nandkumar, and Avinash Kadam. "Role of Naturopathy and Yoga Treatment in the Management of Hypertension." *Complementary Therapies in Clinical Practice* 17.1 (2011): 9-12. Web.

Neff KD. The development and validation of a scale to measure self-compassion Self Identity. 2003.

Oman, D., Shapiro, S. L., Thoresen, C. E., Plante, T. G., & Flinders, T. (2008). Meditation lowers stress and supports forgiveness among college students: A randomized controlled trial. *Journal of American College Health.*

Ornish, Dean. "Can Lifestyle Changes Reverse Coronary Heart Disease?" *2nd International Conference on Nutrition and Fitness, Athens, May 1992: Part II World Review of Nutrition and Dietetics Nutrition and Fitness in Health and Disease* (1993): 38-48. Web

Shapiro, S. L., Brown, K. W., & Biegel, G. M. (2007). Teaching self-care to caregivers: Effects of mindfulness-based stress reduction on the mental health of therapists in training. *Training and Education in Professional Psychology.*

Shirom, A., S. Melamed, S. Toker, I. Shapira, and S. Berliner. "Burnout and Risk of Cardiovascular Disease: The Evidence, Possible Causal Paths, and Promising Research Directions." *PsycEXTRA Dataset* (2005): n. pag. Web.

Williamson, Marianne. *A Return to Love: Reflections on the Principles of a Course in Miracles.* New York: HarperCollins, 1996. Print.

5th chakra

Clift, S.m., and G. Hancox. "The Perceived Benefits of Singing: Findings from Preliminary Surveys of a University College Choral Society." *The Journal of the Royal Society for the Promotion of Health* 121.4 (2001): 248-56. Web.

Kraftsow, Gary. *Yoga for Wellness: Healing with the Timeless Teachings of Viniyoga*. New York: Penguin/Arkana, 1999. Print.

John, P.j., Neha Sharma, Chandra M. Sharma, and Arvind Kankane. "Effectiveness of Yoga Therapy in the Treatment of Migraine Without Aura: A Randomized Controlled Trial." *Headache Headache: The Journal of Head and Face Pain* 47.5 (2007): 654-61. Web.

Singh, Poonam, Bhupinder Singh, Rachna Dave, and Rakhi Udainiya. "The Impact of Yoga upon Female Patients Suffering from Hypothyroidism." *Complementary Therapies in Clinical Practice* 17.3 (2011): 132-34. Web.

Yogitha, Bali, and John Ebnezar. "Effect of Yoga Therapy and Conventional Treatment in the Management of Common Neck Pain - A Comparative Study." *Journal of Yoga & Physical Therapy J Yoga Phys Therapy* 02.02 (2012): n. pag. Web.

Yogitha, Bali, R. Nagarathna, Ebnezar John, and Hr Nagendra. "Complimentary Effect of Yogic Sound Resonance Relaxation Technique in Patients with Common Neck Pain." *International Journal of Yoga Int J Yoga* 3.1 (2010): 18. Web.

6th Chakra

"Biomedical ResearchVol. 29 (2008) No. 5 October P 245-250." *Inward-attention Meditation Increases Parasympathetic Activity: A Study Based on Heart Rate Variability*. N.p., n.d. Web. 10 Nov. 2015.

Birnie K, Speca M, Carlson LE, Exploring self-compassion and empathy in the context of mindfulness-based stress reduction (MBSR). Stress Health. 2010. http://doi.wiley.com/10.1002/smi.1305.

Büssing, Arndt, Thomas Ostermann, Rainer Lüdtke, and Andreas Michalsen. "Effects of Yoga Interventions on Pain and Pain-Associated Disability: A Meta-Analysis." *The Journal of Pain* 13.1 (2012): 1-9. Web.

Gross, Cynthia R., Mary Jo Kreitzer, Maryanne Reilly-Spong, Melanie Wall, Nicole Y. Winbush, Robert Patterson, Mark Mahowald, and Michel Cramer-Bornemann. "Mindfulness-Based Stress Reduction Versus Pharmacotherapy for Chronic Primary Insomnia: A Randomized Controlled Clinical Trial." *EXPLORE: The Journal of Science and Healing*7.2 (2011): 76-87. Web.

Hạnh, Nhất, Mobi Ho, and Dinh Mai. Vo. *The Miracle of Mindfulness: An Introduction to the Practice of Meditation.* Boston: Beacon, 1987. Print.

"Harvard Neuroscientist: Meditation Not Only Reduces Stress, Here's How It Changes Your Brain." *Washington Post.* The Washington Post, n.d. Web. 10 Nov. 2015.

Kabat-Zinn, Jon, Leslie Lipworth, and Robert Burney. "The Clinical Use of Mindfulness Meditation for the Self-regulation of Chronic Pain." *J Behav Med Journal of Behavioral Medicine* 8.2 (1985): 163-90. Web

Keng S-L, Smoski MJ, Robins CJ. Effects of mindfulness on psychological health: a review of empirical studies. Clin Psychol Rev. 2011

Khalsa, Sat Bir S. "Treatment of Chronic Insomnia with Yoga: A Preliminary Study with Sleep?Wake Diaries." *Applied*

Psychophysiology and Biofeedback Appl Psychophysiol Biofeedback 29.4 (2004): 269-78. Web.

Kim, Sang-Dol. "Effects of Yoga Exercises for Headaches: A Systematic Review of Randomized Controlled Trials." *J Phys Ther Sci Journal of Physical Therapy Science* 27.7 (2015): 2377-380. Web.

McDonnell MN, Smith AE, Mackintosh SF. Aerobic exercise to improve cognitive function in adults with neurological disorders: a systematic review. Arch Phys Med Rehab. 2011

Nagendra, Ravindra P., Nirmala Maruthai, and Bindu M. Kutty. "Meditation and Its Regulatory Role on Sleep." *Frontiers in Neurology*. Frontiers Research Foundation, n.d. Web. 10 Nov. 2015.

Satchidananda, and Patañjali. *The Yoga Sutras of Patanjali*. Yogaville, VA: Integral Yoga Publications, 1990. Print.

Sharma, N., S. Sharma, and A. Verma. "Effectiveness of Integrated Yoga Therapy in Treatment of Chronic Migraine: Randomized Controlled Trial." *European Journal of Integrative Medicine* 2.4 (2010): 194. Web.

Tg, Fischer White. "Protocol for a Feasibility Study of Restorative Yoga for Symptom Management in Fibromyalgia." *Journal of Yoga & Physical Therapy J Yoga Phys Ther* 05.02 (2015): n. pag. Web.

7th Chakra

Miller, R. (2006). Your brain on yoga nidra: Questions for Richard Miller KYTA bulletin. http://kripalu.org/jyta_artcl.php?id=265.

Stankovic L. Transforming trauma: a qualitative feasibility study of Integrative Restoration (iRest) Yoga Nidra on combat-related post-traumatic stress disorder. Int J Yoga Ther. 2011.